# THE C.A.M.P. GUIDE TO
# SEX AND THE SINGLE GAY

# Borgo Press Books by VICTOR J. BANIS

# THE C.A.M.P. GUIDE TO SEX AND THE SINGLE GAY

## VICTOR J. BANIS

THE BORGO PRESS

MMXII

THE C.A.M.P. GUIDE TO SEX AND THE SINGLE GAY

FIRST BORGO PRESS EDITION

Published by Wildside Press LLC

www.wildsidebooks.com

# DEDICATION

I am deeply indebted to my friend, Heather, for
all the help she has given me in getting these
early works of mine reissued.

And I am grateful as well to Rob Reginald, for
all his assistance and support.

# CONTENTS

# INTRODUCTION
# TO THE 2012 EDITION

More than any of the other books in the C.A.M.P. collection, I entertained doubts about reissuing this one, for the simple reason that it is the most obviously dated. Of course social niceties have changed greatly since all of the books were originally written, but in the Jackie Holmes adventures there are always stories to distract the reader, and the realities of cooking (*The C.A.M.P. Cookbook*) and astrology (*The C.A.M.P. Guide to Astrology*) have changed hardly at all in the intervening years.

*Sex and the Single Gay* was inspired by the best-selling *Sex and the Single Girl*, written by Helen Gurley Brown of *Cosmopolitan* fame. Like its predecessor, my book offered advice on a wide variety of fronts—furnishing an apartment, for example, cooking, entertaining, styles and—mostly—attracting and seducing men.

Men aren't so much different now from what they were then, but otherwise things have changed on nearly every front. To cite just one example, by 1970, no one batted an eyelash at shoulder-length hair on men, but when I was writing this book only a few years earlier, masculine hair that long was still so rare as to look peculiar. Dancing then was still mostly closed dancing; the frug, the watusi and all those moves commonly seen in dance clubs today were still around the corner. To be sure, in a few clubs you could already see guys shaking their booties, but it was regarded as a bit freaky.

Even the realities of day-to-day gay life have changed. The subterfuge I recommended then will surely seem odd to today's young gay males, who will undoubtedly wonder why the fact of their gay-ness should be concealed from office mates, heterosexual friends, and at straight gatherings. But in those days, though many of us were peeking out of our closets, the gay lifestyle remained perilous—arrests and getting fired from one's job were still realities for many of us, and straight friends and families could and did shun the openly gay. It was still necessary, in other words, to live a more or less secret gay life.

So, why, then, reissue a book that will strike many as out of touch with the gay life of today's readers?

The best reason I can offer is that I think much of what I had to say then is still valid today. Much of the advice—on managing a budget, for instance, or furnishing an apartment still applies (though certainly the prices have changed), and even where it doesn't, there is an even better reason to read—it's funny. Yes, campy funny, but, hey, take another look at the title.

So, in addition to what I offer in the book, I would add this advice—take what you can use, consider the rest of it a window on what life was like for us back then—and in any case, do enjoy, please.

Otherwise, you're missing the point.

—Victor J. Banis

# CHAPTER ONE
## MR. WONDERFUL, THAT'S YOU

It's New Year's Eve, the big night itself. Dressed in your finest, you are (pick one):

1.) at a marvelous party, surrounded by friends. At the stroke of midnight, your handsome date gives you your first kiss of the new year.

2.) drinking alone at a bar, watching the festivities on television and trying to convince yourself it's just a lot of noise.

3.) preparing to jump from the top of your city's highest building.

Did that one scare you? Well, let's try again. Let's suppose you are at a party. Unfortunately, it's been rather dull, and you've just been cornered by a dreary auntie, when into the room walks the most gorgeous hunk of man you've ever seen, and he's absolutely alone. An hour later:

1.) you and Handsome Hunk have managed to escape the dull party together, and are now creating your own excitement.

2.) you are still in the corner with auntie, watching some other guest whisk Handsome Hunk away.

3.) you are applying a splint to the arm that Handsome Hunk broke when you made a pass at him.

All right, just one more before we start tallying up the points. This time you've gone to the opera by yourself. Glancing about, you see some acquaintances of yours in a private box. During the first intermission you send an usher with greetings and a note asking if you may join them:

1.) the usher returns promptly with their message insisting that you join them.

2.) you have received no reply by the next intermission, so you make your way to their box, to find that the door had been nailed shut.

3.) the usher returns and with a smile asks you to follow him; after leading you through endless corridors, he instructs you to go through a certain door. You do so only to find yourself outside the opera house without your ticket stub. Inside, you can still hear the usher laughing.

If your answers to the above little test were all number one, you don't need anything that I have to offer. In fact, you can continue your lovely life, taking satisfaction from the knowledge that I and numerous others loathe you.

On the other hand, maybe you couldn't honestly pick number 1 as an answer for any of the questions. In that case, you most definitely need help—and that's exactly what this book is all about—helping you improve your average. Even if your answers were divided, there's plainly still room for improvement.

It may be a question of developing a little style and grace, or perhaps you've never learned how to approach a desirable man. Whatever the problem, you just might find the answer if you're willing to read further, and try a few suggestions. Considering all that's at stake, that's not asking much.

Of course, maybe you don't regard being attractive, liked, and appealing to men as important. In that case, you deserve to be alone on New Year's Eve, or nursing a broken arm, or standing outside in the rain.

There's no shortage of self-help books available today. I've read most of them myself, sometimes in genuine desperation. And before I go any further, I may as well tell you the truth about myself.

No one has ever been so rash as to tell me I'm beautiful. Furthermore, since my eyesight is good, if anyone did tell me such a thing I'd suspect him of being hopelessly dishonest, mentally deranged, or too drunk to drive.

I am clumsy, rather effeminate, far from brilliant, often quite helpless, nervous, terrified of strangers (to say nothing of high places and the dark), far from wealthy, and I have a genuine talent for putting my foot in my mouth.

At this point I can hear you shrieking that you need my help like you need a dose of you-know-what. Very funny, but let me add a few things.

I've been told by scads of men that I was attractive and/or sexy—and many of those men just weren't gay, not by any accepted definition of the term. Likewise, many of them thought I was sexy enough to find out what "gay" was all about.

I have lots of friends, straight and gay, on all levels of society. Being gay and being effeminate have never been detriments, nor hindered me socially in any way. As for being shy, nervous, or helpless, I've found those items to be assets in many situations.

Without being wealthy, I live well. I just returned from a several-month trip to Europe, and brought back my own car. I have a comfortable apartment, all the clothes I need, and always a sufficient cash reserve to cover those little emergencies that come up.

Bah, humbug, you say? Perhaps you think the answer is witchcraft? Or maybe you admit that this is all possible and fine for me, but how, you ask, does it apply to you? Well, very simply, unless you're a really hopeless case (and I have yet to meet one that hopeless), you can accomplish the same things if you're willing to try. And I'm willing to help. Shall we go on?

There's only one place to begin, and that's with you, the only natural resource you have to work with. And never mind telling me that a silk purse can't be made out of a sow's ear. In the first place, not everyone likes silk purses. Some people go for cowhide, some go for alligator, and some even end up with plastic, so what makes you think that no one would want a sow's-ear purse? Particularly one that's well styled, nicely made, and—here's the most important part—well sold. The first task is making it as desirable as possible, the second is convincing the potential customer that it's what he wants.

Try another little test, if you're still in doubt. Think back to the last time you were with a group of friends in some public place. (I hope it's not that long ago!) Remember their comments about the various men around you. One of them thought one number was just divine, although nobody else in your group agreed. And while the others were drooling over someone in one direction, you were lusting after a sweet young thing that they hadn't given a second glance to.

It's one of the niceties of life that tastes vary. If they didn't, only a small handful of people would make out, and the rest of us would have to suffer. All of which means that, no matter what type you are, there are those somewhere who find your type appealing. You'll have to learn where to find them, and of course, once you have found them, how to convince them that you, of all your type, are particularly appealing.

Don't let the use of the term "type" frighten you either, because it's only a generalization. Actually, you are quite unique, the one and only you in the world. Try though He might, HE'll never be able to find anyone quite as wonderful as you.

That may sound conceited, but it's really not that at all. You see, before you can expect other people to like you, you have to learn to like yourself. Many people, unfortunately, don't. But with the right attitude you can, and should, be the best friend you have. Now think about it, what constitutes a good friend. To begin with, he likes you, and respects you. On the other hand, he's kind but honest in pointing out your shortcomings to you, and helping you to make the most of yourself. That's the kind of friend everyone needs, and the kind of friend you should learn to be to yourself.

Maybe you already like and respect yourself; that makes everything much easier. If you don't, then you'd better start asking yourself why not? Just what is there about you that's not likable? This, of course, is where the honesty becomes essential, because you've got to start right now and take stock of the situation.

Now wait just a minute—you do have to determine what are the faults that need improving, but let's not convince ourselves that you're a walking disaster area. I don't care if you are a troll living under a bridge, you have your good points too. You're a friend to yourself, remember, and no friend is going to spend all of his time gloomily tearing you apart. So, while you're at it, let's make notes of those good points too, because we're going to want to take full advantage of them while we're learning to eliminate or at least play down the others.

All right, to begin with, I'm assuming you're gay. Now that right there is a problem to many people. In our society, it's pretty difficult not to feel self-conscious about it at times, and for some people it can be a really traumatic experience. If, in your case, it's resulted in an existence that is nothing short of a nightmare, then chances are you may need the sort of help I can't give you in this book.

If you are seriously toying with the possibility of suicide, or sealing yourself in an isolated cave, you should talk to a professional. Surprisingly enough, many headshrinkers today don't attempt to "cure" a homosexual, whatever that involves. Rather, they try to help him adjust to himself so that he can lead a happier life.

But let's suppose that things aren't quite that bad for you, in which case maybe you just need to consider a few facts and start using a little common sense.

The homosexual is a lot better off today than he has been in the past. For one thing, just about everyone has faced the fact that he exists, and that he does not possess horns and tails. That helps. For another thing, there's more information available on the subject, for the homosexual who wants to understand a little more about himself. If you're genuinely puzzled by your nature, it won't hurt you to do a little reading. If nothing else, it will soothe your ego to learn that you're not so different from most other people. Homosexual and heterosexual urges exist in most people, in varying degrees.

Nor does being homosexual mean that you have to live your life as an outcast from society. As I said before, I mingle regularly with many non-homosexuals, oftentimes close friends. Once you've learned to accept your homosexuality, and adopted a few rules for social behavior, you can do the same.

As for the other areas in which you need improvement, it's safe to say that there's a solution to nearly every problem. If you're too heavy, or too thin, it's almost certain that you can do something about it—I'll go into this a little further subsequently.

If you're hiding lovely eyes behind owlish glasses, look into contact lenses. If you walk like Carmen Miranda with an overwound spring, fencing lessons or a membership in a gym will help. Voice lessons can do wonders as far as lowering a piercing talk. These are the sort of things which can be detriments for you, and there's just no excuse for not correcting them. In later chapters I'll go into more detail about improving your appearance, and your chances. But by now you should have singled out some of the most pressing shortcomings, and started to work on them right off.

Very well, once you've reached the point where you can start liking yourself, you're ready to see if you can persuade others to like you. There's only one way of accomplishing that goal, and every self-help book, psychiatric journal, or philosophical writing will tell you exactly the same thing—you have to start liking others. You're going to have to be a friend if you want to have friends.

Now that may or may not sound difficult to you, depending upon your attitude toward others around you. But personally, I find it easiest to use the same approach you've been using on yourself—try looking for the good points, not just concentrating on the faults.

There's another little trick that I learned years ago, and which has served me well. It's called Warm Regard and you build it up just as you would a muscle, through practice and exercise.

Start with someone you do like, in fact the most likable person you can think of. When you call him to mind, you'll feel a—well, nice feeling, sort of a glow. Mind you, I'm not referring to lust, or anything so earthy as that. I'm talking about the feeling of liking. And don't kid me that you don't know the difference.

Now, keeping that feeling fixed firmly in your mind, switch to someone else. Be sensible, don't pick the most obnoxious person you can think of, but someone about whom you feel pretty neutral. Transfer your feeling of "liking" to this person. At first it will dim a little, but with practice, you'll find that you really can think nicely about this person.

Of course, you don't stop with mental pictures. The difficult part will be to put this new attitude into practice, the very next time you meet this person. Call to mind your Warm regard, and let it show; be just as friendly toward Mr. Mouse as you always have been toward that most likable person. As I said, this is just like building a muscle—the more you use it, the better it will be. And needless to say, once you've succeeded with this individual, you'll go on to someone else, someone a little more difficult to like. Before you know it, you'll have made friends of some people who were your enemies in the past. Believe me, it's a very nice feeling.

Now I know you can't expect everyone to love you; from time to time, you'll experience some failures, but they aren't too important as long as you're also experiencing some success. If you're not, I'm afraid that the fault can't all lie with the other people.

As for criticism, I know it can occasionally make you sound very witty, but that kind of wit may end up leaving you laughing alone. The best—in fact the only —time to offer criticism is when it's asked for. In that case, be nice about it, be honest, and radiate a lot of Warm Regard.

\* \* \* \* \* \* \*

Well, now things are looking up for you. You're hard at work correcting some of your major shortcomings, and you are rapidly acquiring all sorts of new friends.

But I'm still homosexual, you say. Won't those new friends, the straight ones, change their minds if they find out?

They might, or then again, they might not. There's one important fact in your favor, however—they don't want to find out.

Peculiar though it may seem, people who like you (and by now all sorts of people are beginning to like you) will go far out of their way to avoid admitting the obvious to themselves. They'll do much better than you at inventing excuses for you, and eat their tongues before asking the wrong question. I have seen perfectly sophisticated, otherwise bright people behave like morons rather than recognize the truth about a homosexual friend. Of course, it's your job to make this just as easy as possible for them, which means following a few basic guidelines.

In the first place, you behave naturally. By now I'm sure you've begun eliminating some of the more obvious affectations you've displayed in the past. You weren't born with them, so forget the lame excuse. You learned them, as a child probably, but it's not too late to replace them with better ones.

Now, as I said before, I'm inclined to be effeminate, but don't fool yourself, that's still not the same as being screamy. You don't have to turn yourself into a booted, leather-jacketed oaf, or wander about with a pipe between your teeth. But you can observe some of the men you know, the pleasantly masculine ones, and try learning some of their traits.

The homosexual faces another problem too, the fact that it's too often necessary to be dishonest. Regrettably, this becomes a habit. Many homosexuals call attention to their way of life by putting up too much of a front. For instance—while you're entertaining straight friends, your lover, roommate, or what have you, answers the phone. "For you," he announces, and while you take the call, he goes to the kitchen, where he does not hear the act you are putting on.

"Of course, sexy," you purr into the phone, although it's only your best friend calling. Knowing that he'll understand, you work hard to make it sound as though this were one of many women who pursues you. When it's finished, you give your straight guests a smug grin and explain that it's just an old girl friend.

At this point, your roommate returns to the room and, ignorant of your deception, asks, "What did Charlie want on the phone?" Result, you're left looking like an ass. What's more, your friends certainly will wonder why the deception was considered necessary.

The simplest way to get by with dishonesty is to cover it up with as much of the truth as possible, at the same time keeping the dishonest part to the bare essentials.

Furthermore, you'll have to learn when to be discreet. In other words, you don't rub your straight friend's noses in your business—figuratively speaking, that is. If you run around wearing lace shirts with jeweled buttons, and such garb, you can hardly wonder why straight folk shun your company. After all, they may be forgiving themselves, but they have their friends to consider too, and they don't want to constantly apologize for you.

Tragically, you'll be called on from time to time to make certain sacrifices. The time for cruising is not when you're out with the boys from the office. You might convince them that the sweet young thing you end up leaving with is an old friend, but they're likely to wonder why you didn't recognize him until you saw him in the rest room.

Well, so far we've concentrated mostly on the inside, helping you to improve your outlook and some of your actions. Now of course I realize that you aren't doing all of this just to insure your entry into paradise. Our motives are downright earthy, and I really am getting around to the all-important goal—MAN. But there's still a lot of work to be done.

Remember the Mounties (that's a police outfit, not a sex club) and their motto for getting their men. They do it all with a plan, and they have to go through training first to be certain they're really prepared. So before we send you out on the trail, I want to make sure you have all the right equipment, inside and out, and that you know how to use it. Don't despair, when you end up taking home your prey and properly stuffing him, or mounting him, or whatever you plan, you'll see that it was worth all the effort.

Shall we go on now to the rest of you—the outside?

# CHAPTER TWO
## MIRROR, MIRROR

THIS chapter is going to devote itself to the subject of grooming—now you can put that wash and wear bridal gown back in the closet. I'm not talking about that kind of "grooming." I'm talking about the bare facts—the raw material that is you, and what to do with it.

Good looks, charm and manners are of course no guarantee of success in any endeavor. You can bow, scrape and flatter all you like, but if you look like a slob and have bad breath or a greasy face, you've struck out before the game started. No man wants the spots cleaned off his suit while you talk, and few of them are still using that greasy kid stuff. So let's see what can be done to improve things.

Let's start at the top, with the head (which is just about where we all start, if we're having any kind of fun at all). A good head of hair is one of the most important things I can think of so far as increasing your "plus" quotient. But don't, please, misinterpret my remark. I don't think hair to the shoulders is very attractive unless one prefers women—in which case you're reading the wrong book. And I'll admit that some of those VERY young fellows look downright cute with pageboys— I'm referring to the hair style—but if you're over nineteen, it's time to trim those locks. Little Orphan Agnes is the only one I know of who could get away with never growing up, unless you allow for that other fairy, Peter What's-his-name. The rest of us only make ourselves look increasingly silly as Tinker Belle. Here is a fact to ponder: nothing makes a person look so old as working too hard to look young.

What you do need is an attractive, sensible head of hair, styled correctly for you. And if you haven't yet guessed, I'm leading up to something. Specifically, I'm aiming at those of you who may be a little thin on top. Of course, there are all sorts of funny jokes: So I have thin hair, who wants fat hair? Very funny. And generally unattractive. Granted, that movie actor fairly glistens up there, and I'm one of the countless thousands who get weak in the knees when he comes on-screen. But let's not kid ourselves, he has a lot of other equipment too, the sort that all manages to go perfectly with his bare scalp. I just don't have all of that equipment, and if you do, you're wasting your time reading this book.

In other words, if you are the balding type, run, don't walk, to the nearest salon and get yourself a toupee.

A very close school friend of mine lost his hair prematurely. There was a time when we were both the same age, but I hadn't seen him in years when I paid a visit a year or so ago. Poor friend, he was practically bald and looked a good ten or fifteen years older than me. My first reaction was glee—after all, in the past he had looked so much younger, to my chagrin, and now it was my turn.

Then I remembered our friendship, and my duty. I sat him down and gave him my $10.00 lecture on hair, concluding with the suggestion that he buy some—NOW! Unfortunately, my visit was only a brief one, but I later took up the campaign by mail. Finally, a few months later, I stopped by to visit him again. Lo and behold, my campaign had been successful. He was sporting a headpiece, and he looked positively marvelous. You wouldn't believe what it did for him, to say nothing of those he came in contact with. Before hair, another friend of mine guessed this boy's age at forty; with it, he could quite easily pass for twenty-five. And that, my dear, is quite a difference.

Oh, I know, you say they're expensive. Indeed they are, but no more so than that vacation you've been planning, or that new sofa, and believe me, they'll pay off in far greater dividends. Or maybe you think they look phony—no, not if you get a good one. I'll grant that an expert might be able to spot one, although even that isn't for certain. My friend, for instance, wore his to a barber—who couldn't spot it. And you really can do virtually everything in them—shower, sleep and—well, that other activity we all enjoy.

All right, let's assume you have your own head of hair. Fine, there's still a lot you should know and do about it. First, and this is important—keep it clean and don't plaster it down with a lot of junk that will make you smell like the lamps of China. Hair is hair, and ought to look like it. Many of the women who went in for those bees nests a few years ago just found that they had been stung.

Next task—study your face and try to decide what style you wear best. There is a difference. If you have big ears, for instance, make sure you wear your hair full on the sides. It will help camouflage those milk-pitcher handles.

If you can afford it, which I think most of us can, go to one of those many new hair stylists for men. By now they are available in most cities. I go to one and for $5.00 I get shampooed, massaged, treated, trimmed and styled. I not only look my best when I come out, but I feel positively queenly—and never mind the wise-cracks. Of course, a regular old haircut may cost you 50% less, but then all you get is a regular old haircut. Besides, your chances of meeting your kind of people at a stylist's salon are much better than at the local barbershop. And hair styling is an art in its own right.

Maybe you just can't afford the money, or maybe there isn't a stylist available where you are. In that case, you'll have to use a little common sense and work it out for yourself, with the help of your friends. To make it a little easier for you, I'll offer a few suggestions:

If your face is long, then wear the hair slightly down over the forehead.

If you have a round, fat face, wear your hair higher on top and off the face, with the sides close to the head, to give you that extra height you need.

It's really quite simple if you think about it.

Also, if you're at the time in life where the gray strands are showing through and you don't want them to, by all means go buy one of those do-it-yourself rinses or hair coloring kits. A lot of people love gray temples—I do, for one. But if you don't feel right with the gray, by all means cover it up, it's your hair, and your self-confidence.

Furthermore, I find that, in general, short hair will give you a more youthful look, long hair will make you look more mature.

So much for hair, now let's move down. No, not that far, just to the face. The most important thing you can do to your face is wash it. Don't forget, your skin is covered with pores which exude sweat and oils. When these get clogged with dirt you may have serious problems. Keep it clean, or you'll wreck any and all attempts at good grooming.

Of course, you may already have one of those problems—blackheads. It's not a nice subject, but it's necessary if we're going to have you looking your best. There are many soaps, lotions, and gadgets designed to help you dispose of them—some of them work, some of them don't, but you may want to try a few. Or you can use a more elementary method. Apply a hot towel to your face, just as the barbers do. Let it stay on for 5 or 10 minutes, heating it up again under the hot water tap a few times. Now your pores are opened up; making sure that your hands are well scrubbed, simply squeeze out the little particles of ingrained dirt. Do it gently, to avoid scars. Then, close up the pores you've opened by reversing the process—apply a cold towel to your skin, then put on an astringent, after shave lotion, or cologne. Don't fill the pore up with cream, this will only start another one. Repeat the whole process a couple of times a week, if necessary, to keep your skin clean and glowing.

There is another thing you can do about complexion problems, watch your diet. Sensible dieting has proved more beneficial than all the cosmetics on the market today. If rich foods and pastries set your sebaceous glands (did you ever hear of a less sexy gland?) to churning overtime, try cutting down. And recent experiments have indicated that milk, of all things, may be a prime offender. If you drink a lot of milk, and you have complexion problems, try cutting down on the white stuff.

What about all those other goodies, the creams, lotions, salves, etc., to say nothing of cosmetics. Well, millions of women have spent hundreds of millions of dollars on those items, and you may as well benefit from their experience.

With one or two exceptions, none of them do a thing except give you a nice tingling sensation. Further on in the book I'll touch upon the subject of wrinkles. As for those shadows under the eyes, you can start working on them by getting a little more sleep. Sleep, incidentally, is by far the most effective cosmetic man has yet discovered. Nothing does so much to keep the complexion clear, or the skin lovely and fresh.

You can also cover up those shadows somewhat by applying a little talc to them, but only if you're going out at night. This is certain to be noticeable in daylight, so you'll simply have to suffer along with shadows.

As for make-up—it is next to impossible, I'm afraid, to wear it and not make yourself conspicuous. Oh I know, many queens insist they can apply make-up so skillfully that it can't be detected, but while they're telling me this, I'm trying not to notice their all-too-obvious efforts. Better try to improve upon what Nature gave you—in a natural manner.

Shave, preferably with an electric razor. Know why? Well, I don't have stock in the company, and in fact I don't use an electric razor myself, but a blade razor has a few disadvantages. Did you know that when you shave with a blade you remove a thin layer of skin as well as the beard. I agree that you get a closer, more long-lasting shave, but it does irritate the skin more.

If you simply cannot use an electric razor, then there's one other thing you can do—take a day off. And I do mean off—seal yourself utterly away from the world where no one can see what a slob you are at heart, and don't shave. A day or two off from shaving every few weeks will allow your skin to repair itself somewhat.

Always, always use an after shave cologne, and not just for the sake of smell. It will smooth, soothe, and freshen the face.

I don't go much for talc, except as I mentioned it

before. And it's perfect for soothing the neck when the laundry puts too much starch in your shirt collar. It's also useful for cleaning, but I'll touch on that in the section on clothing.

Of course, some people prefer to keep their shaving to a minimum, by sporting whiskers. Personally I don't go for them, and if you're growing a beard with the thought in mind that it will make you appear more masculine, don't kid yourself. But, if you really want one, you'll have to use the same sort of common sense with it that you did with your hair style. For instance, a full chin beard will broaden a long face. A pointed beard makes the face look longer, while a rounded goatee covers weak or large chins. A mustache and beard help diminish a large nose. Men with thick upper lips can benefit from a thick mustache, and thin upper lips are helped by thin mustaches.

Insofar as eyebrows are concerned, don't be afraid to pluck them if they're too unruly or odd-shaped. If they cover up the bridge of the nose, by all means separate them with a good pair of tweezers.

There's one other area of hair about the face that you just cannot justify on any grounds—clip those nostrils regularly. You can buy special scissors, separately or in a manicure set, for just that purpose.

Now we come to one of the most important aspects of good grooming—smell. Two eminent psychiatrists wrote an article recently entitled "The Smell of Love." They hinted at the fact that women prefer the good masculine body odor, which a friend of mine interpreted to mean that men aren't supposed to bathe.

Now I really don't think that's what they meant at all, but they did make a lot of sense in that masculine odors can be the sexiest thing about the man. Now let's face it, if we really liked men to smell like women we certainly wouldn't be bothering too much with men, would we? On the other hand, a good cologne or deodorant can make or break your chances. How would you like to go to one of Katy Winters' parties, knowing how many smelly friends she has?

Here again you'll have to decide what smells good on you and what you should stay away from. Too much lime on some people just increases the oiliness of their skin and exudes an unpleasant aroma which I hate standing next to, let alone sleeping with. Now don't get me wrong in that you have to go out and get the most expensive colognes you can find. I'm merely saying find the one that suits you. You, above all others, should know the type you are.

If you're six feet four inches tall and built like a football player, of course you don't want to smell like a Japanese Geisha with a lot of musk and jasmine. If you're slight and petite, okay, get some lime or lemon scents, or a slight trace of oleander or violets. You can afford it.

I have a very close friend who owns more colognes than I have ever seen laid out on bathroom shelves and counter tops. And know what? With all his expense and bother the best thing on him is the $1.50 bottle of Old Spice he buys at the super drug store. He's far from the $1.50 type, but that just happens to be the best scent on his particular type skin. Even when he tells people what it is, they think he is joking.

So know yourself and then shop for that which suits you. And don't feel foolish sampling various types. When at the counter just rub a couple of them on different parts of the skin and sniff. You'll be able to tell which is best for you. When you've picked out the one, wear it, and I mean wear it right. Don't mix scents, which just loses the benefit of all. And don't change scents once you've found the right one. You want a scent that will say you whenever he smells it, even if it's on someone else. If he can picture you every time he smells Snuff (the cologne, not the real stuff), and you have sprinkled a drop on the gift wrapping paper of the birthday gift you sent him, he's certain to thank you with exceptional warmth.

Know where to wear it too. Behind the ears, contrary to what everyone thinks, it is wasted. Put it on the temples, at the V where the neck and collarbone meet, at the wrists and—are you ready for this?—behind the knees. Those are the points where it will last, and radiate all sorts of messages to him throughout the evening—and night.

Also, and always—and I mean always—wear a deodorant and use a bad-breath combatant regularly, like at least twice a day, just to be sure. In the former case, there are all kinds—some that don't smell at all, some that match your cologne. They vary in effectiveness with the body chemistry of individuals, so find the one that is most effective for you. As for bad-breath, there are countless mouthwashes and mints. Many salesman, by the way, swear by antacid tablets, such as Rolaids—most breath problems start in the stomach. And if you have a real problem, see a dentist for advice. It may be an indication of more serious trouble, although I can't think of anything more serious than scaring men away.

Believe it or not, statisticians have proved that within the next few years sales of men's toiletries will far outnumber those of women if the current trend continues. Keep it up. Everything possible is now available to the man, such as hand creams, hair sprays, perfumes—you name it, they market it.

Dry skin problems can be easily remedied by simply applying cold cream or even Vaseline on your face before going to bed. If you use Vaseline for other purposes, incidentally, I'd recommend two separate jars. If your hands get too dry and scaly do the same thing to them. Once a week treatment should be sufficient, but use nightly treatments if you're very dry, and watch out for particularly cold or windy weather.

For the oily skinned among you, frequent washing with soap and water and applying an astringent two or three times a day will help, as will talcum powder.

Don't overlook the finger and toenails. Keep them trimmed and well filed. Never taper them, keep them short and even, and above all, clean. And never, never, never apply polish of any kind. I don't care what your straight friends do—even Esquire is against polish on men. There are creams, too, for rough hangnails and cuticle problems. Look into them if you are afflicted with such problems.

Your body in general is my next topic of conversation. We're all inclined to be lazy, and consequently so much you'll have to do depends upon the sort of shape you're in. And if you're absolutely out of shape, I'd suggest you see a doctor, or consider a gymnasium.

Let's hope, however, that things aren't that far gone. In that case, a few simple rules will work wonders.

To begin with, the next time you have to go to the market, which is several blocks away, please don't walk to the carport and drag out the convertible. Walk—it's still one of the best exercises available. And if the load of groceries on the way back is a little too heavy for that long trek, good—make two trips. That'll do you twice as much good.

A friend of mine has an executive type job, private office and all that. I paid him a call one day and noticed that everything in the office was almost inconvenient to the desk he occupied. "Why?" I asked. "It's simple," he told me. "I get my exercise that way. If I need something I have to get up for it. It helps keep my backside from spreading out."

You may be interested in knowing that his backside was sufficiently "unspread" to make it one of the most sought-after in the city.

Another very simple exercise you can use while taking Rover for a walk or just strolling along the street. Carry something you can drop on the sidewalk now and then, just to make yourself stoop over and pick it up. It helps that advancing waistline more than you think, and there are other benefits as well.

You may not know it, but exercising will make you less tired. You see, certain acids have a tendency to build up in the body, particularly at the joints, and as these acids are passed into the bloodstream, they create that "tired" feeling often attributed to not taking Geritol. By exercising, you burn up these acids. For that reason, one airline executive recommends the above exercise for long flights—that is, dropping a pencil or something so you have to bend down for it. Of course, that's only recommended for flights in a plane. It could be risky on a broomstick.

Everyone hates to exercise, I know. But if you happen to live with someone, you'll find an exercise program in which everyone participates easier to keep up than one you do alone. Anything you do alone is really not as much fun as having a partner, don't you agree? Of course you do, that's why you're reading this.

Diets, naturally, are another source of pain and discomfort, but another necessary evil. Serious overweight or underweight problems, as I said before, should be handled by a professional. But if your problem is only an advancing tummy or the like, a few sensible habits will make the difference between being lovely or ludicrous.

If you have to go to that beer bar every night, then for goodness sake make sure you account for the calorie consumption by cutting down on the sweets and stuff you normally have with dinner. And you can also investigate the caloric count in such things as vodka and tonic (180 calories) versus Scotch and soda (90 calories), or martinis (170 calories) versus Manhattans (235 calories). Get the picture? A Rob Roy will only cost you 110 of those nasty things, but a zombie, weighing in at 520, isn't worth it.

Just to give you a few ideas, I prepared a little list to indicate some of the danger areas:

## BEVERAGES:

black coffee...NONE!
w/cream...25
cream & sugar...55
tea (naked)...NONE!
milk...165
ale...100
beer...100
sweet cocktails...250
dry cocktails...90
highballs...150
liqueurs...80 to 90
whisky (a jigger)...110 to 150
sweet wine (1 glass)...130
dry wine (1 glass)...95

## BREAD:

white...65 (one slice)
rye...70

biscuit...100
English muffin...130
Danish pastries...120
Saltine (double)...40

## DESERTS:

chocolate layer cake...400
pound cake...115
cookies...110 to 125 each

Now, good habits, remember, are a prerequisite, so start now and don't flinch. Take that extra few minutes every time you go out or before you settle down for an evening of television, to work on your grooming. You'll thank me, and yourself, I guarantee. And even if you do wind up spending the entire evening alone, you'll feel a whole lot better sending and smelling your nice, fresh, clean self into that trundle bed.

# CHAPTER THREE
## GILDING THE LILY

WELL, by this time we should have you pretty well straightened out—don't let that term scare you—on the inside, and outside we've made you about as lovely as possible. However, since we simply can't send you out on the job with all that naked loveliness, we're going to have to do something about clothing you.

Let's start by putting down the book, walking over to the mirror, and taking a long, cold look. Oh well, you say, who expects me to look my best when I'm merely sitting home reading a book?

Don't kid yourself. You know as well as I do that the best opportunities come at the least expected times. What are you going to do if that maddeningly attractive gas man knocks at the door and your appearance is enough to scare him out of his tubes? So, before we go any further, and if your attire is what I think it is, go dress properly for an evening at home. If the slacks are too snug for just sitting around, then you shouldn't be wearing them anyway. And speaking of pants, which happens to be a subject we all think about a lot, let's start there.

Your first consideration in trousers, your own that is, should be your own naked, lovely self. Please don't pour yourself into something that's five sizes too small just so that lovely virility you like so much to exhibit turns out looking more like a ready-to-be-lanced tumor. Remember, a sense of mystery is always more intriguing.

Take careful note of your waistline. If it happens to be the same size as your hips, you are not only in trouble, but you didn't pay attention during the last chapter. In that case, before and during your weight losing period, try to find some inexpensive, trim but not tight, trousers that will not accentuate your over weight.

If you are short and stocky, please never wear such things as patterns or plaids. Stripes are fine, but keep them very vague. Nothing too prominent. There's nothing worse than a fat woman in a floral print or a brilliant chartreuse suit.

In other words, examine your shape. You should know what makes you look good and if the body is bad, don't bring more attention to its uneven proportions by draping it in eye-catching materials. You may be of the opinion that nice bright colors will call attention to your face which, with good grooming, is very satisfactory. Well, if you think that, I want to ask a question.

When you're sitting in your favorite haunt and some dream person walks through the door, what do you notice first? His face you say, right? WRONG. If the face is quite lovely and the rest of him is a round, or oval, 229 pounds, I very much doubt if you will think the face nice enough to take between your crisp white sheets. Unless, of course, you prefer 229-pound men. If you do, well your evening is made. I'll say no more.

Likewise take your shape into consideration before going overboard on those new, marvelous mod (or maude if you prefer) styles so lovely to look at on those delightfully trim young boys. Again, if you happen to be a delightfully trim young boy, then by all means, be my guest, go hog wild.

All right, let's begin at the beginning. You've determined the type of shape you have; if not, stand in front of the mirror and, with a lipstick or some such thing, draw a rough outline of yourself. With that accomplished, let's cover the basic body types, and some general rules for dressing them. I'm ignoring the body beautifuls, they can get away with wearing almost anything and still look like body beautiful.

STOCKY, BULKY TYPE: In your own best interests, stay away from the wild, way-out patterns. No prints, plaids, or checks. You'll want to stay with medium or dark colors, as light colors will only tend to make you look even heavier. Small up-and-down weave effects are fine, but please don't ever contemplate the heavy, nubby fabrics like tweeds and such. Very light material will crease too easily, so avoid it. Keep the clothes trim but not too tight. Never wear tapered legs and if you wear them cuffless it will make your legs appear a little longer. Stay away from the cut-away front type jacket and please, no wide lapels; on the other hand, don't wear extremely skimpy lapels either. A good moderate width is very definitely your best bet.

Try to avoid flaps on the jacket pockets and don't dwell under the impression that vests will make you look slimmer and hide your wrinkled shirt front. The vest will only bind you in the more, so if it came with the suit, leave it in the closet. It's not for you.

Low, long-point shirt collars will look best on you. Again, please avoid splashy sports shirts and brilliant ties, and above all else never wear a bow tie. Of course, if you are wearing a tux, it's another story altogether. Then I fear you'll have to stick to convention even though it won't suit you at all.

Some of you will disagree with my next remark, but here goes anyway. Wear medium to large jewelry. Regardless of what people say, your bulk will blend with the size of your jewelry. Now I'm expecting you to continue using a little common sense. Leave that five carat diamond pinky ring at home when you go cruising, but do wear it to the opera. And don't worry when your friends tell you it's ostentatious—of course it is!

THE THIN TYPE: If you happen to fall into the thin category, you can almost read through the preceding paragraph dedicated to the bulky type and just turn around and do exactly the opposite of what I recommended there. Your suit and/or sports coat will give you that extra weighty look you so need if you will select patterns like plaids or checks. Above all else avoid the vertical stripes. You'll wind up having people stringing bean plants around your ankles.

So far as color is concerned, you're lucky. Depending upon your skin coloration and such, you can wear anything, light, medium or dark, although the light colors will add weight.

Try to get as much weight into your fabrics as possible. Stay away from those articles of apparel that will pull you into a long straight line. A jacket with a slight trace of shoulder padding and a hint of waist suppression will give you a broader, heavier look. As I said before, if you want to look like that bean-pole, go ahead and wear that real short length jacket; you'll get your wish.

Unlike the bulky types mentioned previously, you can by all means wear that vest—the fancier the better. If you like double breasted suits or blazers, by all means get them. They're really your best bet.

Taper your trousers and always cuff them if you are tall and thin. If you're short and thin, leave the cuffs off. Wide shirt collars will broaden your face, and don't be afraid of a pattern in your tie. Sports shirts can well be either plain or patterned, whichever you think preferable.

IF YOU'RE SHORT: Your first and prime consideration will be all those outfits that make you look taller.

You can achieve this by adhering to one overall color or variation thereof. In other words, don't wear a black jacket and light gray slacks. The contrast is too definite and will tend to cut you down. But a black jacket and very dark gray or navy blue slacks are fine. See what I mean? Your best bet, in fact, will be the all black outfit.

Avoid anything that will shorten you, like double breasted blazers, flaps on pockets, wide lapels, cuffed trouser legs. Vertical designs in patterns are good, but please, in moderation. Short jackets will make your legs appear longer, as will tapered legs on your trousers. For people such as yourself, the legs should always be more tapered than they are ready made— have a tailor do it for you.

When wearing a tie be sure it's the narrow variety, and your shirt collars can be tab, regular spread, or long pointed. Jewelry will definitely be of the small variety. And don't be tempted by those expensive, elevator shoes. They just make you uncomfortable and don't do all that much. Use that money elsewhere.

YOU LUCKY TALL ONES: vertical stripes are out for you, unless you want to look nine feet tall. You too should stick to solid colors, but you're very fortunate in that you can actually wear just about anything. Plaids, checks, tweeds, bulky fabrics, they'll all suit you well.

Pay attention to anything horizontal—I don't mean those you find in your bed, that comes in a later chapter. I'm referring to double breasted jackets, vests or suits, flaps on your pockets, wide-spread collars and striped ties—stay away from them all.

Your jackets should fit loosely and be a nice medium length with wide, lower cut lapels. Just be sensible about your accessories. Don't wear anything that will exaggerate your height.

* * * * * * *

Well, that covers the basics as far as body types. Now let's take a look at color, which is another area where many people fall down in selecting a wardrobe. We just can't all wear the same shades, and that striking color that looks so great on your sister may look awful on you.

Virtually everyone and anyone can wear the color blue. It goes will all complexions. All hair coloring, all color eyes, with perhaps one exception. Redheads can wear it, but I wouldn't recommend it. Redheads should stick to grays and browns, and green, of course, but be careful in the selection of shades.

Occasion will sometimes dictate the shade you wear. For instance, please don't wear a powder blue suit to an evening affair, unless of course it's a powder blue dinner jacket. Then, of course, you'd wear it only to a formal dinner, and in the summertime.

If your eyes are light, then choose a dark shade or medium shade of blue to enhance their color. If you have vivid blue eyes, powder blue is spectacular. All one shade of blue is a bore. Almost any color except tan will mix well with blue. Green may also prove a bit hard to handle, but it can be worn if chosen carefully. Generally, pick blues and greens in different values—that is, a dark blue with a pale green, or vice versa. Or stick to the soft, grayed greens. Be careful also with browns. For the most part, you'll want a pale or medium blue, and a dark brown.

Men with black, brown, red or silver hair can definitely wear grays. Blonds would be wise to keep to medium or dark shades of gray. Accents for gray are many—white, blue, pink, pale yellow, pale olive. A lot of people dislike maroon and gray, although I've seen it worn quite successfully.

As for brown (watch it, buster)—brown-haired men can wear any shade of brown they like, but blonds pretty well have to stick to medium or dark shades. Men with red hair should stick with the reddish-brown shades, while charcoal brown is lovely for black-haired men. Sallow complexions should avoid olive or golden browns.

Accents with brown are white, tan, yellow, pale olive and the true greens. Pink and red striped shirts look great with those lovely gray-brown colors. light gray and blue also can work well.

Olive, outside of martini talk, is a very flattering color for you brown-haired devils. Blonds are also safe in the same category, if they stick to the lighter shades. If you have a pale complexion, olive may unfortunately leave you mistaken for the corpse at a funeral. As for accents, try white, tan, gray, olive and yellow, and of course blue. And if you're the real daring type, try pink, or a nice red-striped shirt with the darker shade of olive.

I began this chapter with the recommendation that you look in the mirror, and I assume you took my advice. I do hope that you're not now dressed in black silk suit, shirt, tie and highly polished patent leather shoes. Knowing what to wear is one thing, knowing where to wear it is another. Later on I'll discuss the size of your wardrobe, but right now I'd like to talk about places and people.

Where are you right now, in bed? Well then you definitely should be nude, or nearly so. Pajamas are fine, but they are restricting and in my opinion, a waste of money. If you have any sort of company at all, they'll spend more time under or alongside the bed than on it—your pajamas, I mean, not the company. The only time your company should be under the bed is when more company arrives, unexpectedly, and you fear a scene. And if you're not having any nighttime company at all, just who are you wearing those pajamas for? Invest that money in some other wardrobe items that pay off better.

The same is true of robes—they're lovely, I suppose, but save them for gift hints. Anyway, I think a man is much sexier walking out of a shower with a towel around him. And towels can be removed so much more quickly.

We started at scratch, so to speak, with nudity, so let's pursue that just a little further. Nudity has its advantages. Now I'm not advocating nudism, which to my mind is not particularly sexy, but you can use nudity to save on your wardrobe. Ann Landers touched upon the subject in one of her columns, and was startled by the number of letters she received from housewives who stated that they did their housework in the raw. It does sound economical, but if you decide on this, better have something handy to slip into before you answer the door.

When lounging around the house, which I assume you're doing at present, a nice clean pair of jeans, preferably pressed and neat, loafers or sneakers, socks, and a simple T-shirt are fine. If you happen to have a nice cashmere sweater, I have a personal fetish for wearing a cashmere sweater with nothing else touching the upper half of my body. I know an awful lot of visitors who share a similar taste.

If you're going out to the local haunt, your choice of clothes will depend upon the type of haunt, although of course whatever the choice, they'll be clean and pressed. If it's only a beer joint, jeans will be fine, the same ones you are wearing to lounge around the house. And if they don't look nice enough to wear outside, they aren't nice enough to lounge around the house either, remember that gas man. Toss them and go nude about the house.

If it's coolish when you're going out, of course you'll have a nice, casual jacket or sweater. As for draping that sweater over the shoulders, you might be mistaken for Whistler's Mother in her shawl. Sweaters and jackets are equipped with sleeves so they will fit on your arms.

If your body is a little thin, or not yet all it should be, work harder at it, and in the meantime be sure to wear the jacket. A little camouflage helps.

For dinner out, a shirt and tie with a sports jacket or

suit. If it's a really casual spot, then an open neck dress shirt, sans tie, is fine. This outfit, by the by, will see you safely in and out of most bars, and it gives you that crisp, just out of the laundry look, even if you don't work in a laundry.

There will always be those times when you should dress—dinner, the theater, and the like. This means a suit—no dark sports jacket and dark slacks. You need THAT suit, black or dark blue, and stylish, without being too extreme. Get a good one, at one of the better stores, even if it costs a week's salary. Wear it not too often, and care for it properly, to make it last.

All right, having started on wardrobes, I may as well discuss the things you do need. The dark suit, as I've said, is a must. Silk is your best bet. Mohair cracks, so watch out for it. Next come slacks, remembering the colors, etc., that are right for you. One or two pair will suffice. For myself, I love those wash and wear things on the market, the good brands.

You'll need a sports jacket, one that will blend color-wise with you and your slacks. Don't go out and buy that wild maroon and black striped blazer you've been admiring either, unless you can afford a closetful of jackets. If you only have one or two, everyone, including yourself, will soon be tired of that wild number.

You need a sweater or two, good ones that will wear well. They may be a little expensive, but you can save part of the money with sports shirts. Here you can be a little silly. If you buy that mad, mad shirt in the bargain basement, or on sale, it won't hurt too much if you get tired of it after a few wearings. Don't get too carried away, however, and find that you haven't money left for anything else. And don't buy those shirts just because they're on sale. They should still be your color and style.

Lots of ties are a ridiculous extravagance. Three or four are all you need, if chosen with care. The widths and colors should flatter you, and go with your wardrobe.

Handkerchiefs should be plain white and always neatly pressed. Nothing is more disappointing than the lovely creature at the bar who, of necessity, reaches for his handkerchief and pulls out a crinkled mess that may have come from Heaven alone knows where, and how long ago. It doesn't make me want to take him home and do his laundry for him either. I just feel that he's lazy, and look further. Of course, if he's too too gorgeous, I wouldn't let a crinkly handkerchief come between us.

A raincoat or topcoat is probably essential. If you live in a warm climate, one of those black numbers with a zip-in lining will suffice, and can even be worn for dressy occasions.

Shoes, of course, but not a closet full. Have one pair for dress, always polished and on shoe trees, and don't wear them for anything but dress occasions.

You need a few items of jewelry, but remember that one nice set will be more impressive, and probably cheaper, than a drawer full of junk.

That's about all that you really need in the way of a

wardrobe. For example, my own wardrobe, and I do a lot of traveling, mixing, etc., includes: the black suit, a conservative olive suit, a mildly striped sports jacket that mixes with the slacks (I have other sports jackets but they were gifts, so they don't count; anyway, I usually end up wearing the same one or two), two pair of wash and wear slacks, one sweater, one pair dress shoes, one pair "ordinary" shoes, one pair loafers, a dozen pair of socks, three ties, a raincoat, and some shirts. So I'm not putting you on. If you're contemplating spending a fortune on clothes above and beyond that basic wardrobe, save the money instead. Later I'll have places for you to invest it.

The most important thing you can learn about your wardrobe is the care of it. Keep dry cleaning to a minimum, it's death on most fabrics. Brush suits, etc., often, and steam press them yourself. Always hang them up, on shaped hangers. For stubborn spots—use talcum powder on oily spots, such as spaghetti splashings. Sprinkle it on, let it dry, then brush it off. Repeat as often as necessary. Incidentally, the best clothes brush is still the cheap, ordinary whisk broom. For other spots, use a cleaning fluid, or cold water. Soap, and warm water, tend to "set" spots. If they remain, then rush them at once to a cleaner, and describe the nature of the spot.

Never put jackets over chairs, or shoes by the fire. Don't load your pockets with heavy objects which will stretch them out of shape.

Starch is murder on shirts. The more starch the

shorter the life of the shirt. Incidentally, there are wash and wear shirts, including dress shirts, that do work. Wings makes an Endura Press, and there's a more expensive Permanent Press Arrow. Remember that these are best if machine washed and dried. In the sports shirt line, H.I.S. makes a fine permanent press number.

Entire books could be written on the subjects we've covered so far—several books have been, in fact. But if you'll keep all of these suggestions in mind, you won't have too many problems. Our task is not to turn you into a clothes horse, but to help you look your very best for our campaign. And, with that campaign in mind, we have other things to discuss. You're about to begin the post-graduate work, on the way to becoming an expert.

# CHAPTER FOUR
## ABOUT VENUS AND OTHER FLY TRAPS

WELL, so far we've covered quite a bit of ground. We're well on our way to creating a new you, starting with a new outlook on life. We've done everything possible to improve your looks, and learned how to make the most of your appearance with careful grooming, and proper dress.

At this point, we've just got to stop and be honest with ourselves—that's important in a friend, remember, and we're both trying to be your friend.

Everyone can't be beautiful. I know it hurts; believe me, I've suffered the pain many times. Unfortunately, very few people really qualify to be called beautiful, and even then others don't always agree as to who qualifies—personally, I don't care for violet eyes.

On the other hand, we don't have to be like the famous, and homely comedienne who insists that she decided, at age twelve, on inner beauty. Fortunately, beauty just is not an essential in the man-catching game. Isn't that a relief! What you need is sex appeal.

Oh, dear, I thought that would produce a groan.

Well, just be quiet for a moment or two, and think of the people who are famous for their appeal, the movie stars and such. Taken at face value, few of them are really beautiful. In fact, some of them are downright homely, aren't they? So you see, there's hope for little old you.

Again, just like looks and types, what appeals to one man won't appeal to another—thank Heaven. However, I'm going to offer a few suggestions for making yourself appealing to most people, most of the time. Some of the suggestions are my own, some are frankly borrowed from those famous sexpots we were discussing earlier. Let me warn you of one thing, however. Given the right man, the right mood, and a mysterious chain of circumstances that no one can predict, and you might be unbearably sexy with a stream of blood on your face—but that doesn't mean you should take a razor to your forehead every time you have a date with him—unless he's really a nut, and, in my estimation, not a desirable.

First and foremost, think sexy. No one knows why this works, but thinking sexy thoughts and feeling sexy will do more than anything else to get him thinking the same way. As I told you before, lots of men have told me I was sexy, and I've already admitted that I'm no beauty. I rely on sexy thoughts. When I can't make myself think or feel sexy, all of my other efforts are wasted.

One expert has pointed out that hair is sexy. I agree to a point. I think clean hair in particular is sexy. On the other hand, those impossible creations held in place with glue and baling wire are just not sexy in my opinion. Keep it clean, and simple, and if you need a hairspray to manage your tresses, try the Alberto products. They hold my hair, which is like weak corn silk, so I'm certain they'll hold yours, and they comb out nicely without leaving you chewing gum for hair.

Padding, for the most part, is not sexy. As I said in the chapter on clothing, certain types need a little padding at the shoulders, but don't overdo it. And there are, in case you haven't discovered them, pads for just about everything else.

Personally I think that the real thing is going to look even smaller if your date has had his eye on what proved to be a "false front." As for artificial fannies—well, I have a friend who wears one, along with occasional padding on his legs. Unfortunately, he can't wear all that when he gets down to bare facts, and as a result, he looks like an entirely different, and less appealing, person.

Being neat and well groomed, which by now you've mastered, is very sexy too, but here again you can go overboard. If you recoil in horror because you see a stray hair on his lapel, he's liable to take his strays and leave.

Being pleasant is sexy, but don't smile so much that you look like a moron. And learn to sit quietly, without fidgeting and scooting around. That's sexy.

Never talk too much, which is very unsexy—but talking about the things that most interest him can be sexy. Of course, talking about yourself is not sexy, while being a little mysterious is. One of the unsexiest things I can think of is talking about other men. If he refers to them, inform him innocently that he's the first one you've ever met. Brazen, but sexy.

The right clothes, as I've mentioned before, are sexy. If they are baggy, or too tight, they aren't sexy at all, just vulgar. New clothes make me feel sexy (and feeling sexy is sexiest of all, remember?). Even new shoes make me feel sexy, but then sometimes I feel sexiest when I'm barefoot. Remember Ava Gardner in that movie?

As a matter of fact, no clothes can be sexy, too. Now I'm not advocating nudism, which generally tends to become unsexy. But an unexpected glimpse of you, or part of you, can be very sexy. When you're stepping out of a shower, for instance.

Colors are sexy, the right colors for you. I'll go into your apartment, in a manner of speaking, later but why shouldn't you pick out the colors there the same way you picked out the colors for your wardrobe, to flatter you—and weaken him?

Weather is sexy, No, of course you can't control it, but you can take advantage of it. Some spring nights were just created for a stroll, and the evening will do more to further your schemes than all of my suggestions. Likewise for autumn, with falling leaves and all that. And nothing can be cozier than being alone with him, inside, when it's awful outside.

Food can be sexy, when you've fixed that lovely meal

for him—and I'll help you with that later.

Being alone can be sexy—he'll be far more interested when he calls and finds you alone than if you're surrounded by a pack. Solitude in general is sexy—cliché—he travels fastest who travels alone. You need friends, but don't make yourself just another member of the gang—there may be some among them whom he won't want to court, and he may feel that he has to take them too if he wants you.

Problems can be sexy, particularly listening to his with a sympathetic ear. Yours will rarely be sexy, unless he can help by doing something you know he enjoys. If, for instance, he's a nut about cars, and you ask him to help you shop for one. Money problems are never sexy. Not even his!

Money, however, is sexy, particularly enough money to do the things you enjoy doing. But I'm saving money for a later chapter.

Wearing glasses can be sexy—now don't ask me why, but a person looks more like he's really reading, or working, when he's wearing glasses. Glasses, when he's trying to kiss you, will be unsexy if they get in the way.

Reading can be sexy in various ways. Reading aloud to him will be sexy if he's the right type. And reading to improve yourself or your knowledge is very sexy.

Working, too, can be sexy—particularly if he's your boss, or in the same office where he can appreciate your efforts. Anyway, working is sexy if it gives you a chance to express the real you—and afford all these other sexy things.

Intelligence is sexy—now I don't mean explaining Einstein's theory and such, but good common sense, and a quick wit. But being too smart can be dreadfully unsexy, when he starts thinking you're smarter than he is.

Sleeping can be sexy, if you don't snore, and keep your mouth closed. Sleeping when he's talking is not sexy.

Scents are sexy—the scent of his favorite food cooking in your kitchen, or that cologne you've finally picked out. By the way, have you considered a matching soap. I'm still not convinced that it makes you smell any better, but it always makes me feel awfully sexy. As a matter of fact, being clean is sexy, but like neatness, it can be overdone. Smelling at least vaguely like a real human is also sexy. Being sweaty at the right time, such as after that game of tennis, is sexy. Being sweaty other times is unsexy.

Having energy is sexy, the energy to help him paint his living room, or keep up with him when others poop out. Bounding about with energy when he's pooped may not be very sexy.

Fireplaces are sexy—flames in general are sexy, such as candles. Of course, burning his trousers is not sexy, nor is a roomful of smoke from the fireplace. Dim lights are sexy too, but not if he's trying to read, or play cards. And having a headache from dim lights, or anything else, is unsexy.

In fact, being sick is just about as unsexy as you can

get. Never be seen when you're sick in bed—unless it's by the handsome new doctor you've discovered, and you feel well enough to be sexy. If you don't feel well enough to be sexy, you really are sick—may as well let him send you to the hospital, you may spot a few interesting patients. And if he's not a handsome doctor, or at least interesting, you're also sick. Look for another doctor.

Music is very sexy. Vocal music is less sexy, except for French vocal music. The "Prelude" and "Leibestod" from Tristan und Isolde, in an instrumental version, is about the sexiest music I know.

A low voice is sexy—lower yours, but making him strain to hear you is not sexy. Telephone calls are sexy, whether he's calling you, or you're calling him. Being awakened in the middle of the night, except by a nudge, is not sexy.

Dancing is sexy. I'm not talking about those gyrations in vogue today, unless you're less than twenty-five. Over twenty-five, you simply can't look sexy doing them.

I was recently in a club where men were dancing together—at least a hundred men. I could scarcely keep my eyes off one man. Although he was probably nearly forty, he was anyone's match for sex appeal, with gray temples, haunting eyes, and classic profile. My heart broke when he went to the dance floor with a young thing. All traces of sex appeal disappeared as he flailed his arms, shook his hips like Gilda Grey, and stomped his big feet. He returned to the bar bathed in sweat, his hair flopping over his forehead, panting with exertion. I turned my attention to someone else.

Try a tango, however, or a rhumba, and see if that isn't sexy. Stepping on his feet, or trying a dance that he can't do, or you can't do, is not sexy. Dancing better than he does is not very sexy either.

There are very few things sexier than liking men—I don't mean just being hot for them, although one can't help that sometimes. I mean really liking them, and showing it. It's very sexy to remember his birthday or special occasions, and working late with your boss is sexy, as well as good business. And taking him a cup of coffee at his desk when you know he's too busy to get away for some will convince him you're awfully sexy. So will pitching in for that extra chore, without grumbling. Grumbling is not sexy.

Cocktails are sexy, and even though getting drunk is not sexy, it is sometimes useful.

Cruising is sexy...

Now I've done it. I have a feeling I'd better stop right here and tell you all about cruising, because it's more than sexy, it's positively essential.

\* \* \* \* \* \*

I don't know how you define cruising—to many, unfortunately, it just means running down the street after a handsome number, or leering like the Big Bad Wolf from under Grandma's bonnet. To me it's how you let him know that you think he's special, and you're interested, or even that you might be interested, or you aren't interested, but you could be if he were.

Does that sound confusing? All right, let's take an example.

There you are and there, suddenly, he is. He may notice you, or he may not, it doesn't matter—cruising has nothing to do with how he reacts to it. Anyway, you see him, and you feel something—mild curiosity, desire, hope, or just plain carnal lust—but a reaction. That, in its most elementary form, is cruising, and whatever you do about that feeling is cruising too. Whether you wink, stare, introduce yourself, ask around about him, send him anonymous letters, or attack him with a club—it's cruising.

Here's your first lesson. If you're out right now, start at once; if not, try it the very next time you're out in public. Look for a man—now some people call that cruising, but to me that's prowling. Cruising is when you spot one. Anyway, pick out a nice one and look at him. Wait until he looks back then, peering straight into his eyes, let yourself melt slightly, and look away. Count to twenty five, but slowly—never rush cruising—and look at him again. Picture a great big question mark in your mind, and try to make it show in your eyes. Then look away again. Very good. You're cruising.

Next lesson. This time you're talking to a man. If you were really good at the above lesson, it may be the same one, but if not, it can be just about anyone. This is only practice, so it won't hurt if you're not serious about marrying him. Look straight into his eyes as though you were watching the sexiest show you've ever seen. Be there an earthquake, flood, or police raid, don't look away for an instant. Breathe deeply, let your mind join with his for a second.

You see, you're cruising again. Isn't it fun? And this particular method has been used by every famous sex symbol since the one with the pyramid and the big asp. Think about it, isn't it sexy when someone is hanging on to your every word, instead of looking all about the room and only half paying attention?

Oh, yes, you have to learn to listen. Never interrupt him, even if some jealous queen approaches from behind you and sets fire to your coiffure. He is talking, and you're interested in him, so you're also interested in whatever he has to say.

When he is telling a story, or a joke, pay very close attention. Cry when he gets to the sad part, laugh at the punch line, and swear aloud angrily (the one place where you can interrupt) when he tells you how badly his boss treated him.

If you aren't cruising at least two hours a day, something is wrong. There are men everywhere, and you can use the practice. Cruising is sexy. Cruise that cop who gives you a ticket (maybe I'll get around to telling you some of the adventures that has promoted), cruise the elevator operator in your building, cruise the young man selling magazine subscriptions, and the checkout man at the supermarket. You never know when someone will cruise back, and anyway practice makes perfect.

There's one other point that I want to bring out before

I leave this subject—being cruised. When someone else cruises you, or makes a pass, he's paying you the nicest compliment possible. He's saying that you are sexy, at least to him. Be nice about it, even if he's two feet tall and green-tinted. In time, I'll tell you how to discourage such advances, but for the moment just remember to be nice, and grateful for the compliment. If he thinks you're sexy, so will someone else.

Anyway, now there's three of us—him, me, and yourself—who think you're sexy. How's that for progress?

# CHAPTER FIVE
## BELLES AND BILLS

JUST think, a short time before you were a drab, lonely creature and now you're a new person altogether—reeking with personality, scrubbed clean, dressed to the fours, and fairly pawing the ground for a chance to get all those men I've promised you.

Hold on—I'm sorry to say that we aren't ready yet. There are still things to be discussed before I can turn you loose on them. Why go to the battle half-armed, when in only a few more pages you can be really prepared. Remember the Boy Scout motto—or is it the Marine Corps'?

It takes money to be sexy. And there's no point in wailing and crying "foul." It's one of the rules of the game, and you can't ignore it unless you want to lose.

Don't get me wrong, I'm not saying you have to be wealthy. That would probably attract a few males, but if you think about the yo-yos who hang around the wealthy aunties you know, you'll soon realize they aren't what you're after. You can do better and with less money.

But you do need some money. More important, you

need to know how to use what you've got. It's possible to be genuinely elegant on a few pesos a month. Some people can't achieve that result with millions, because they don't know what to do with it. So let's take a look at your finances, and learn a little about using them, shall we?

To begin with, you've got to face up to the facts about your financial situation. If it's really hopeless, you need a professional, just as you would with severe physical disorders. Money Mess is one of the worst diseases I can think of, but it's curable. You won't cure it by hiding from creditors, any more than you'll cure measles by staying away from red spots.

The most drastic cure is bankruptcy. If there's really no hope for straightening things out, you might want to consider the possibility. An accountant, or even an attorney, will be able to advise you fully, and fill you in on the costs. Oh, yes, it's a paradox, but it takes money to file bankruptcy.

In most states, bankruptcy is not the only alternative available to Money Mess sufferers. For instance, it's usually possible to have a court appointed administrator take over your finances. What he'll do, in short, is collect all of your earnings, except a very small allowance on which you are to live. With the money he takes from you, he juggles your accounts and divides it up so everyone gets a little, but regularly. This, of course, means living close to the belt for a while, but providing you don't keep up your bad spending habits.

Finally, if your will is strong and your need desperate,

you can attempt to do exactly the same thing yourself, but you simply cannot violate the rules.

You'll start by listing all of your expenses and bills, what it takes for rent, for food, and essentials. Also, every single penny that you owe to everyone anywhere in the world. Then you write down what you make a week, or however you're paid. Ghastly, hum?

Let's take a hypothetical situation. You bring home $350.00 a month. Rent, utility bills, food, and the bare essentials account for $185.00, leaving $165.00 to work with. Your car payment is $65.00, your charge account is $20.00, another charge is $10.00, your stereo payment is $30.00, the necessary treatments at the doctor's add up to $40.00 a month, insurance is another $25.00, and the hair stylist I sold you on accounts for $5.00 more.

That doesn't work out too well. As a matter of fact, it leaves you $60.00 short, and that's not allowing for any goodies.

All right, you'll have to find some place to whittle. Are the treatments really necessary? Could you get by with two visits a month instead of four? Is it possible to refinance any of those payments, or all of them? It can't hurt to try on all of them. And it might be necessary to skip the stylist for a few months.

One thing is an absolute necessity, you have to stop spending. Forget the charge accounts, and don't add another cent to them. The rates they charge are exorbitant anyway. With your balances, you're spending more on interest each year than you are on merchandise.

If your loans or any of those payments are with a bank, they may permit you to pay only the interest for a couple of months. Here's the vital part, however. You use that money to pay off the bills that you can, starting with those that have the smallest balances. For instance, let's say the charge accounts stand at $200.00 and $150.00 respectively. That's dreadful. But, if the bank will permit you to pay only the interest on your auto loan for two months, that gives you almost $120.00 to apply to the smaller of the two charge accounts. And if you can stall the doctor for a month, that charge account is gone altogether, and a $10.00 a month payment is eliminated. Then you start on the other one.

It takes time, patience, and a strong will, but eventually you can eliminate all of the charges and installment payments. Even with the car still as high, assuming you can't get it financed, that leaves you $30.00 to the good each month.

All right, so much for desperate measures. Let's assume that your financial situation is not quite so drastic, or that you've managed, after a few month's work, to straighten it up. Now how do you go about making your money work for you, the way it should?

There's no shortage of books on managing a budget. Some of them are sheer nonsense, and some of them contain some genuinely helpful suggestions. You might read a few, and see if you can get some ideas.

There's one point on which they'll all agree, and which I will insist on also. That's a savings account.

Spare me the arguments, it's a necessity. Regardless of how poor you are, you can manage to save two dollars out of your weekly salary. Have it taken out by the payroll department, or deposit it when you're at the bank cashing your check, and before you can spend it. In a year, even at that small rate, you've saved $104.00 plus interest. That's not even mentioning all the other savings I'm going to help you make. For the present, you can tuck them into the bank, in addition to (not in place of) your weekly $2.00

The next thing to do is to find ways to save. If you'll spend just a day or two making a note of every penny you spend, you'll find a few places to save yourself. Those five cent candy bars, chewing gum, extra coffee on your break, and such will add up to maybe a dollar a week, in some cases much more. All right, into the bank with it, and never mind telling me you can't afford it, you've been spending it haven't you? That gives us $156.00 in the bank a year, plus interest.

The next step is in the same vein, but more direct. You have to determine which of the things that you're spending your money for are essentials, and which are non-essential. This sounds easy, but it isn't. You have to be brutally honest, and totally ruthless with yourself. If you can convince yourself that an extension telephone is essential, you aren't being honest enough. It isn't. Walking to the next room will be good for you, in fact—remember the section on exercise.

A basic telephone is regrettably essential in our schemes. But there are ways you can trim the expense.

In the first place, if you haven't already made the mistake, a color telephone is not essential. You can hear and talk as well in black and white. Nor do you need a Princess phone, a Prince phone, a Continental phone, or any other variation of the basic theme.

If you live in a large city, calls to outlying areas will cost you toll charges or message units, or some such thing. Watch those calls. Keep a three minute egg timer by the phone, to warn of passing seconds.

Long distance is a luxury you can't afford. Save it for the family at Christmas, in lieu of a gift. Or a genuine, no-nonsense-about-it emergency. Otherwise, write letters. And you don't need to send them airmail either. Outside of an emergency, Thursday will be as good as Tuesday for its arrival. Unless he is out of town, and it's to him. Then send it airmail.

Writers and certain professional people find it necessary to buy newspapers and magazines of various sorts. You don't. Buying the newspaper every day accounts for another $44.50 a year, when you could be reading the paper at the coffee shop, and magazines at the library, or the doctor's office. Adding that to your bank account gives us $220.00, plus interest. See how it's adding up, and we've scarcely begun, Of course, when you have the extension phone removed, you'll add what you were paying for that to your savings account too.

You need stockings, as another example, but you do not need a crateful. A dozen pair of stockings in black or dark brown are plenty for anybody. And what about underwear, is it really essential? Shorts cost a dollar a pair and up, which is a lot of money, and not to mention T-shirts. All right, if you think they're essential, why not limit yourself to a minimum and wash them every other evening? And you can increase the mileage by not wearing them when you're at home.

Next to that black suit, which is essential, they're practically the most expensive item in your wardrobe, so treat them as such.

You do need certain grooming aids, and niceties for the bathroom. But you do not need a shelf full of junk. Bath salts, room deodorizers, bowl brushes, and such make fine gifts to receive. Keep a list of these items, and when people ask what you'd like for birthday or Christmas, offer them a copy. Never mind if they think you're crazy asking for a toilet brush. Take a peek into your bankbook, and remind yourself of your goals.

You do need bedding, for instance, but a few items of linen and a blanket are all, plus a spread. Electric blankets and mattresses that vibrate are nonsense that you can't afford.

Cocktails are essential, as you'll learn in the section on entertaining, but you don't need Chivas Regal, or Beefeaters Gin.

In other words, you want to stop spending your money on junk and concentrate on the important, essential items, the ones that have real utility value, or pay off in genuine pleasure—the latter, in my book, means making men happy.

The next step is just as important. You pay the minimum price for everything, short of stealing it.

What are you paying for that shaving cream that I admitted was essential? Is there another brand that sells for less? Buy the other brand and see if it doesn't work just as well. Of course it does, convince yourself! What about toilet paper? You don't need two colors, or flowers, or reproductions of Grandma Moses' finest. I'll admit there's a limit here—you don't know the meaning of roughing it until you run across some of the tissues I've tried. In Spain, where they really live cheap, they provide what we refer to as brown wrapping paper. But you can shop for the cheapest brand that is still soft enough to be acceptable.

This goes for other household staples and gadgets, assuming that they are necessary at all. Kleenex or similar grand tissues, for example, are not essential. Use a handkerchief, which can be washed and used again. Why flush all that money down the drain? And shop for these staples in an outlet store, not that swanky shop you feel so nice being seen in. You won't feel nice being seen in debtor's prison.

All right, by eliminating a box of face tissue every month, cutting two cents off toilet tissue, and four cents off shaving cream, we've added $5.00 to that yearly savings. That's how it's done.

What about stationery? Of course you have to write letters, but isn't there paper at your office? Use that, and write letters on your coffee break. Personally, I save writing paper and cards from hotels and motels when I'm traveling. It saves me money, and provides interesting stationary—besides, it reminds those friends who snicker about my Christmas list that I can afford to travel.

Charge accounts, as I mentioned before, are murder, and should only be used for an absolute, unavoidable emergency. Buying records when they're on sale is not an emergency. However, if you discover at the last minute that it's his birthday, and you have no cash on hand, and can't manage to borrow it from anyone, that's an emergency. A gift for his birthday, incidentally, is an essential, but that doesn't mean it has to be a new Jaguar roadster, or something of that sort. It can be a book, or a tie, or even something you've done yourself, such as fixing him a special dinner. In my opinion, the latter sounds far more interesting than dropping a box (cardboard variety) into a mail slot.

I mentioned borrowing—that's reserved for emergencies, and lending is reserved only for double emergencies—make that triple. If he's really stunning, make it a single and a half, but don't be shy about asking for it back, and don't let him make a habit of it.

You may want to investigate using the long form on your income tax. It's sometimes worth investing in a tax man.

A car is an area of big dispute. Personally, I don't think one is necessary. Later, when you can afford to pay cash for one, that may be a different matter. Now I know, if you live in a big city like Los Angeles, you're going to start screaming about the difficulties of getting around. All right, let's look at the facts.

A short while back, I leased a new convertible, at a

special rate, thanks to connections. Even at the special rate, it cost me $90.00 a month to get it into my possession. Added to that was $10.00 a month garage rental. That's $1,200.00 a year, plus another $136.00 for insurance, And that's not even taking into consideration the necessary expenses involved in driving it, such as gasoline, oil, and maintenance.

If you'll use even a fraction of your brain power, you'll quickly see that that is quite a few rides in a taxicab, and more bus rides than I feel like counting. If you combine buses and cabs, which I used to do, you can manage quite well—a bus ride going, and a cab returning when, hopefully, I was accompanied, or else just too tired to feel like standing at a bus stop.

If you're going out with a sister, why pay for the most expensive seats, or go to the plush restaurants. You can see the movie from further back, at much less expense. And there's just no reason for you to be eating out by yourself. Take your lunch, or eat a large breakfast and keep lunch to a bare minimum.

You can save money too when you're shopping to eat at home. There are terribly expensive cuts of meat, and slightly less expensive cuts of meat. Save the best ones for when he's coming. Never throw a scrap of food away. There are all sorts of stews you can make for yourself with those leftovers that you accumulate. One bean may add just the right flavor to a pot of homemade soup, and you should know that the bone from the roast, even picked clean, will contribute to a fine broth.

Prepared foods are more expensive. Learn to boil your own Brussels sprouts, which is healthier anyway. And always buy items that are in season. Fresh tomatoes in the winter are very expensive anywhere in the north. Save them for special occasions.

Wash your own sweaters and shirts. As I've said, cleaning is hard on clothes, and by now you've learned to brush and steam clean them. Add the cleaning charges to your savings account.

Your bank probably has a special account for checking, which means it costs less if you write fewer checks. By all means, write fewer checks, and take the cheaper account.

If you pay the utilities at your apartment, never leave a light burning unnecessarily. Watch water and gas too. If there's a drippy faucet, beg the landlord to have it repaired, pronto. Don't use electric appliances for jobs that could as well be done by hand, such as opening a can or beating an egg yolk. In cold weather, close your drapes to save heating bills.

It's not easy being a pinch-penny. You'll have to cut out those mad spending sprees you used to go on, stop trying to impress your sister with your wealth (which they never believed in anyway), suffer the occasional snickers and sneers of those who think you've flipped your wig, and spend at least twice the amount of time shopping that you spent in the past. Is it worth it? Well, take a look in your closet—chances are there's a jacket, shirt, or sweater in there that you bought on one of those impulse shopping sprees, one that you've worn only once or twice since then. Just think, that money could have gone toward something useful. And in the refrigerator is a bottle of East Indian fermented clay wine which intrigued you in the gourmet shop, but proved undrinkable. In its place, you could have had a fine brandy to serve him.

In the long run, he's the big factor. When you can afford to groom yourself the way you should be groomed, dress yourself the way you should be dressed, entertain him and others the way they should be entertained, and live the way you should live, your chances of catching him are at least tripled. He is the reward you're working toward. Once you've got him, I think you'll agree he was worth a cheaper brand of shaving cream.

# CHAPTER SIX
## IN YOUR LITTLE LOVE NEST

PICTURE this, if you will: You've worked on the man of your dreams for positively weeks. Progress, even if it has been slow, has at least been steady. He's at your apartment, his resistance weakened with cocktails, drowsily stuffed with that scrumptious dinner you prepared. The music is sweet, and so is he. This, you tell yourself jubilantly as you move in for the kill, is the night. You can virtually see the love words forming on his lips. At that moment, the door bursts open, and your roommate sweeps into the room, followed by what appears to be, by virtue of numbers, the entire cast from a Cecil B. spectacular. Do you:

1.) Hide in a closet with your date;

2.) Persuade your date to entertain the group with his rendition of the mating call of the titmouse;

3.) Suggest a reenactment of the Little Big Horn massacre, with you playing all the Indian parts?

Try another one. The rain outside would be enough to drive Noah to his ark, but inside it's cozy and warm. He's there, and at his offer to start a fire in the fireplace you proudly produce the marshmallows you've been saving for just this occasion. Having rid yourselves of the clothes that got wet when you were caught in the downpour, you settle yourselves on the bearskin. At this precise second, the telephone rings.

Your roommate is calling from far up in the mountains, where he has just allowed your car to go over a cliff. Not only does he need rescuing, but your car will need to be towed out before it is swept away in the mudslides that have started. Do you:

1.) Leave your date alone, hoping that he'll keep all of the fires going for the three hours you'll be gone;

2.) Announce in a feminine, businesslike voice that the connection has been broken and all telephone lines are down at least a month;

3.) Suggest that your roommate hold a piece of metal over his head, to see what the lightning will do?

Are you beginning to get the picture? All of your efforts will be to no avail if you are not free to carry them out. I've heard some people say that they had roommates and the freedom they needed. Personally, I find this believable only if the roommate spends his time hanging by his feet in the closet, and comes out only during the full moon. Now don't misunderstand me, you can't have too many friends, whom you will from time to time entertain, and who will reciprocate. But if you have your heart set on snaring a man, or several men, you need an apartment of your own.

What do you need, specifically, in the way of an

apartment? To a degree, that depends upon you, and your budget. A small apartment of your own is better than a shared mansion. Furthermore, it will cost less to furnish a small apartment—I'll pursue this further in a little bit, and give you some suggestions for saving those all-important pennies.

Most advisors agree that the neighborhood is not terribly important. It's you, and your apartment, that he's coming to see, not your neighbors. If he's the type who is easily impressed by fancy neighborhoods, you can go ahead and try to impress him, but that will probably mean a more expensive car, all sorts of priceless gifts, and an extra mink to use as a car robe.

My personal advice is to chuck that one, and look for one who's more interested in you than your purse.

You will look for an apartment that fits you and your budget, one that lends itself to decorating possibilities, and affords a certain amount of privacy. Solid walls aid in the latter, and best stay away from pool apartments, where all the tenants tend to live as one big happy family. Unless, of course, you've found a few interesting prospects among the tenants in the building you're considering.

Decorating is essentially a matter of taste; your apartment should express you and your personality. Remember, however, that you want the men in your life to be comfortable in it also. Too much fuss, too many doilies, and chairs that look like they will collapse when sat on, tend to make most men uncomfortable. If you genuinely prefer period pieces, there are periods that are more masculine in feeling than others. And why not add a few pieces that don't match. As a matter of fact, my decorator friends are in unusually solid agreement that a roomful of furniture pieces all looking exactly alike is pretty poor decorating.

Decorating an apartment can be a costly venture. It's a sad fact that if you fill it with things from the dime store, it may end up looking like a dime store department. However, there are some things that will help you save money and achieve the results you want—among them are skill, imagination, taste, and time.

Skill you just can't expect to go out and acquire overnight. If you've already got a decorating degree from Vassar, you may as well skip this whole chapter. On the other hand, it's quite possible you have a decorator friend, and he might be coaxed, over a second martini, to give you a few pointers. If you haven't such a friend, or he can't be coaxed (some friend!), there are still experts waiting to serve you. For one thing, there are those people in the department and furniture stores. Oftentimes there'll be someone on hand to offer you some decorating advice free of charge.

Last but not least, you can read—I know that for a fact, because there are no pictures in this book. And there are plenty of books and magazines dedicated to decorating. Read some of them, look at the pictures, and especially watch for rooms that are similar to yours, of arrangements and color schemes that seem particularly pleasing to you.

Imagination is likewise hard to acquire, but the same

sort of reading I just suggested, plus of course this book, may help along the imagination you've already got but aren't using—likewise for taste.

Time, surprisingly, is one of your best allies. Researchers insist that the shopper who, probably because his money is limited, must take a long time to shop, and look around for the best prices, etc., usually makes a better purchase. Impulse purchases are more often than not ghastly mistakes, so if you can't afford to furnish your apartment in one expensive trip as soon as you've signed the lease, you're probably better off.

Probably the best place to start decorating your little castle is with the color scheme. Generally speaking, you'll probably want light colored, unobtrusive walls, which will make your subsequent decorating easier. Bright colors and bold patterns will be more effective if used in smaller quantities for accents, or in an area that is used more briefly, such as the bathroom, or a dressing room if the apartment has one.

Of course, you have a right to your taste, but I'm warning you that most men will feel smothered in a very tiny room papered with red cabbage roses. You'll be safer with walls that are beige, off white, etc. If the apartment is already painted in purple, or papered with frolicking clowns, start by having a tantrum for the benefit of the landlord. Cry, hold your breath, fall into a faint, and whatever, but do try to convince him that he should paint the walls for you. He may not, in which case you'll simply have to do it yourself.

Shop at one of those great big stores specializing

in paint and home improvement goodies. Ask the salesman for advice, and don't hesitate to take the paint chips home and see how they look with your light and what have you. It will be easier if you get the paint guaranteed to cover in one coat—except for the kitchen, where you'll probably want something easier to clean.

The floors are another consideration. If you're lucky, they'll be carpeted, which reduces noise, heating costs, and in general adds to a room's charm. If it's not carpeted, you'll have to make do with area rugs. Don't forget to put one in front of a fireplace if you have one. Also necessary is one by the bed—you don't want him to get cold feet at that point—and a small one for the bath. Finally, if you are wealthy enough (and convinced you're going to be in the apartment for a while), you may want to install carpeting yourself. If you do, do this before you start the other decorating— it's easier to match draperies to rugs than vice versa. For the most part, carpets should be in darker shades, to give a room a solid feeling.

Drapes, too, may be included. If not, set out with a sample of your wall color and carpeting (never rely on your memory of these colors) and start shopping. Don't, incidentally, forget to take along the measurements.

If your room is small and you want to make it look a little larger, stick to drapes that match or blend with the wall color. If you have a number of separate windows, try covering them all with a wall of draperies.

All right, now we're ready to tackle the actual furnishing of the place. Up until now you've presumably slept in a sleeping bag and used packing crates for tables. Take heart, the worst is past.

You might possibly have rented a furnished apartment. By and large, I'm not in favor of this idea. Most of them are furnished with sheer junk, and with the difference in price between furnished and unfurnished apartments, sometimes as much as fifty dollars a month, you could soon own your own.

This is where imagination becomes of major importance. All of those books and magazines you've been devouring are just filled with do-it-yourself ideas for the one on a budget. Many of them just don't work, but don't give up hope. And never mind telling me how lousy you are at that sort of project—you couldn't possibly be less skilled at carpentry than I am, and that doesn't stop me from trying—oftentimes quite successfully.

One of the sexiest apartments I can think of belongs to a friend of mine with very little money to spend. For all practical purposes, it's only one room. Off that, of course, there's a bath, and in the other direction, a small kitchen with a dining area. I'm assuming you got a bath with yours, and something in the way of cooking facilities, if it was only one of those closest arrangements. Big kitchens are nice, but not necessary.

Starting with nothing, my friend added velvet drapes, which he made himself—an ambitious project, I'll have to admit, but the results were certainly worth it. Not satisfied with merely those folds of fabric, he added a cornice board, which he padded and covered himself.

Next investment was a sofa, and this was where he used his money, all he could spare. In other words, he got a lovely one that looks just chic as a sofa and makes out into a perfectly comfortable bed for two.

With a lot of looking around, he found a big, nicely made but unfinished cabinet, in which he installs stereo components as he can afford to add them, and a beat up portable television he bought second hand. Needless to say, he finished the cabinet himself, using one of the kits available at paint stores, or even Sears. Again, it's largely a matter of taking your time, and of course following the instructions.

He added some simple, inexpensive occasional tables, and managed to find, at a Salvation Army store, some old lamps. Gilt paint on the bases and shades covered in Contact paper transformed them into very attractive items.

Finally, he tracked down a chair in a used furniture store and replaced the upholstered seat himself. Then he painted the wood, which was most of it. When the paint was dry, he painted it again in black, and then used turpentine on a rag to wipe off most of the black, to give it an antique appearance.

For the dining area, the best he could do was a round metal table. This, however, he camouflaged neatly by making a round tablecloth to hang to the floor—he made this out of felt to match the color of the drapes, and added fringe at the edge.

With a few accessories stuck about, he had created a very stylish, very comfortable room—or actually, apartment—and the entire operation cost him less than $1,000.00.

If you're really pinched, you might be able to find a sofa in a used furniture store too, and refurbish it. Likewise, you can tuck the stereo components into a closet, and leave just the speakers visible—they're available in nice wooden cases.

There are no ends to the ways in which, by spending a little time and effort, you can save a lot of cash, and reap big rewards. The local lumber company will cut three-quarter inch plywood to your specified size for table tops. To these you'll add the legs, available at a hardware store. The top can be finished in count- less ways—with Contact paper, for instance, or even with picture puzzles. Chances are the lumber company will also cut the molding to put on the edges (although you'll have to finish it yourself). With a coat of bar-top, available at a paint store, the surface will be reasonably safe from burns, spilled drinks, and the like.

Another friend uses the heavy foil gift wrapping paper for many decorating jobs. He first crumples it into a ball, crushing it tightly. Then, very carefully, he unwraps it again, and uses it to cover folding screens, fireplace hoods, and all sorts of things (consider this for a lampshade). Once he has it glued on, he takes some black paint on a rag and wipes this across the crinkled surface, to create a veined effect, just like hammered gold.

Needless to say, unpainted furnishings can save you quite a bit. Virtually every city has one store that specializes in these pieces—dressers, occasional tables, cabinets, etc. It's more work, but I'm presuming you have more energy to squander than money.

Don't overlook the possibility of greenery. Fresh growing things add something to an apartment, and if you can't afford a great big rubber plant, then buy something smaller and raise it yourself.

You'll need one or two nice items to give your room that extra something—a big lamp, if you can afford it, or even a couple of huge, expensive ash trays.

Other than sofas, lamps, and dressers, what exactly will you need for your apartment? Well, you can make do for the present without a lot of occasional chairs, by utilizing those big floor pillows. In any event, if there's only one sofa for the both of you to sit on, he'll have to stay close, which isn't such a terrible thing.

You do need ash trays—even if you don't smoke, he may. Don't worry about a lighter, you can serve the same purpose if you fill a glass dish with matches from everywhere you go, adding a pack or two of those very decorative things from the gift shop.

Music is very nearly essential to your schemes, so a phonograph will be needed, but as I've hinted before, you can buy components, starting with essentials and adding to them as you have money to spare. You don't need an entire closet full of records—a few nice albums of romantic background music, and maybe one or two of your own or his favorite.

You'll probably want a television set, to watch that special show with him, or to entertain yourself when you just don't feel like going out, but it doesn't have to be the biggest colorest, expensivest thing in the store.

Candles. I suppose romances have flourished without flickering flames, but I've never known candles to slow any down. They'll lessen the shock of that dinner which, regrettably, burned, take years off your appearance at a fraction of what it would cost for a face lift, and add a romantic touch that just can't be accomplished any other way.

A telephone, unfortunately, is necessary. I know that they're dreadful people to deal with, and expensive, but if he can reach someone else for a date by phone, and has to contact you by carrier pigeon, he may take the easy way out.

Books do a lot for a room, and by some process of magic appeal to men, even men who haven't read anything since glancing over one of McGuffey's Readers. You can buy these at a used book store, making it a point to add some nice ones with attractive covers. Fill out the shelf with paperbacks or gift books that you've hinted for to your friends and received as gifts. It isn't necessary, but you might want to make a point of picking up a few that you're really interested in reading. Someday you may be sick in bed.

Pictures, likewise, work magic. This is one area in which a sale can be worthwhile. If nothing else, buy some cheap prints or travel posters, or clip something from a calendar. Add a cheap frame and, if you can manage it, do a whole wall in this manner.

That, surprisingly enough, just about takes care of the living room. If it's a combination living room-bedroom, you're saved some additional expense.

If you have a separate bedroom, it goes without saying you'll need a bed—only one. And that dresser you purchased unfinished and which came out so lovely. You'll need a light, preferably three-way, which means you have the light to read in bed, or you can make it dimmer for—well, other things.

Bedding, of course, but not an entire trunkful. A few sheets and pillowcases will suffice. I suppose a blanket is necessary, although it seems to me a drab way to keep warm, and a bedspread, which need not be custom made.

For the bathroom, by all means have big, fluffy towels, and the necessary sanitary facilities. Add one of those large brandy snifters from the dime store, and fill it with the soap you snitch from motels, or a package of fancy soap. However, have some real soap on hand too. Most men feel just plain silly in a shower clutching a rosebud to their armpits.

For the kitchen, you will need plates, glasses and the like, but you can serve a stunning dinner without Limoges china. The same goes for pots and pans. Few cooking utensils work as well as a plain cast iron skillet, unglamorous though it may appear.

There, you see, it wasn't such a lot, was it? Mind you, there will always be those extras you'll want to add as you go along, but no one expects you to move into an apartment one day and have everything in it the next day that one could ever need or desire. Start with the essentials, those which are really necessary for functional purposes, or which give your apartment the comfortable, easy to be in atmosphere that men love. It's very hard to love an apartment, and not care a little for the occupant.

# CHAPTER SEVEN
## FUN AND GAMES

BY NOW I suppose you're convinced that I'm never going to let you get to the important things, like getting a man for yourself. Well, indeed I am, but there are valid reasons for my delay. By now I have not the slightest doubt about your ability to interest a man in you, and if all you have in mind is a fast roll in the hay with the first available, then I'd suggest you spend this evening accomplishing just that.

However, tomorrow evening, with some of your natural urges thus attended to, you may want to return to this volume. You see, I'm trying to prepare you for something a little more than a fast roll. And, at the same time, I'm thinking in terms of those men who are just a little less available, the ones you have to work on and convince a little—in other words, the prizes.

Prizes are sometimes, although not usually, available for those little quickies I mentioned above. But even if you find one who is that democratic in his thinking, it just seems to me a waste of a real prize not to take further advantage of all that he has to offer— and that means an affair, possibly even something longer than that.

Sex isn't quite as important to a prize, for the simple reason that he usually has all of it available that he needs. When you invite a prize home, he expects more. And that's what I'm getting ready now to prepare you for—entertaining.

Entertaining can be any number of varied and various events. It can mean simply having a few sisters in for tea and biscuits, or it can involve throwing a really fancy ball. One of the nicest forms of entertaining is the dinner for two—you and him.

You'll have to entertain occasionally for the mere sake of repaying invitations. Some people don't abide by this rule, but most hosts, myself included, soon catch on to this and stop inviting guests of that sort.

In addition, a party is a good way to meet people, even your own party. It's perfectly proper to suggest that your invited guests bring a friend, or there may be a casual acquaintance you've only recently made; inviting him to your party will break the ice for a possible relationship between the two of you.

All right, so you're convinced that entertaining is necessary. Stop quivering and trembling, it really isn't all that difficult, at least not for a person with your charm and sex appeal.

Since your first entertaining schemes will probably center around him, I'll start with dinner for two. His sex appeal notwithstanding, it will probably be easier on your nerves than a large affair. Of course, things may progress between the two of you to the point when, almost any evening, he might be on hand for dinner. For this reason, I think it's a good idea to be prepared, by having a few things in the pantry especially for such emergencies.

Too often the possibility of a really romantic mood is lost for the necessity of trudging down to the local sandwich shop to fill your stomachs. Better to open a few cans and rely upon candlelight and music for flavoring.

I shouldn't have to warn you, on the other hand, that there are some men who take advantage of that kind of hospitality. If it turns out that he's on hand every day at meal time, drop a polite hint or two that it's time for him to repay by taking you out somewhere, and not the local sandwich shop. If he doesn't take the hint, start shopping for someone more appreciative.

My task would be made much easier if I knew that you were a Cordon Bleu graduate, or the equivalent. This may shatter you, but I must be honest, I am not a great chef. Don't panic, though—I am a good cook. Many satisfied, and thus weakened, men have voiced their approval of my talents, even my cooking talents. So if you honestly can't cook, I'll do what I can to help you.

If by any chance you are calling to mind the lovely feasts displayed in various women's magazines, all looking too lovely to eat, you may as well forget all about them right now. Most of them are too something to eat; anyway, so far as I have ever been able to determine, none of them can be done.

You will certainly want to invest in a cookbook, since I can't do much more than a few suggestions in this one chapter. The question of which cookbook, however, is a big one. After years of cooking, I am still often stumped by the directions in certain cookbooks. And there are some that, frankly, require a different attitude toward food than the one which I possess. Personally if I must begin a lobster dish by stabbing the poor creature between the eyes, and remember to watch out for his tail when I cut it off, because it keeps going, I doubt that I would find the dish very tasty when it was prepared.

The James Beard Cookbook, available in paperback form, is one of the best I've found, so far as telling you how to prepare some really superb dishes in a no nonsense manner. The Esquire cookbook, too, is specifically aimed at the inexperienced chef. There's another one, a veritable gem that concentrates on plain solid American cooking and provides just about all the basic information anyone could want, but one regrettably you won't find in your neighborhood bookstore. The name of it is (hang on to your hat) Granddaughter's Inglenook Cookbook, and it's printed by the Brethren Press, Elgin, Illinois.

While you're busy shopping for that cookbook, however, you might want to try out the following dinner suggestion. For the main course you'll need:

2 to 4 pork chops about 1½ inches thick. Some people
    will regard 1 each as sufficient, but most men eat
    more heartily than that. Have the butcher cut pockets

in them for stuffing—never mind, dear, he'll know what you mean.

About 3 cups, maybe a little more, of dry bread cubes. You can buy these packaged for stuffing, or cut up some bread in cubes and dry them yourself in the oven.

2-3 tablespoons of chopped onion.

¼ cup melted butter or margarine

¼ teaspoon poultry seasoning—you'll find this on the spice rack at your supermarket.

1 can cream of mushroom soup with ⅓ cup water.

Start by putting just a little oil in a skillet, heating it, and adding the chops. Cook them until they are browned (that's a legitimate cooking term denoting color) on both sides. Then remove them from the fire and set them aside for a few minutes to cool.

Meanwhile, find a very large bowl in which to dump the bread cubes, adding the onion, melted butter, poultry seasoning, and ¼ cup water. Mix them together—the easiest way is with your clean hands. Then take the chops, when they're cool enough, and tuck a little of the stuffing into the pocket of each one. Place in a baking dish, and scatter the rest of the stuffing about the chops.

Mix the mushroom soup with ⅓ cup of water, and pour this over the chops. Now they're ready for the oven, which you've preheated for 10 minutes, to a temperature of 350. Bake them for one hour, and a little longer won't hurt, as you want them nice and tender.

What about the rest of the meal? Well, there are

infinite possibilities, but let's keep this as simple as possible. If you can find some minted pears in the canned fruit section of your store, chill and serve them on a bed of lettuce, after you've grated a little cheese over them. If you can't find minted pears, then buy a can of plain Bartlett pears, and a package of lime Jell-O. Prepare the Jell-O well in advance, according to the package instructions—but use about ¼ cup less water than called for. Add the pears, drained, to the Jell-O and allow this to set. Serve it as a salad.

With the chops themselves, a can of corn, either cream style or whole kernel will be fine. Now I know I told you that packaged and pre-prepared foods were more expensive, but for your initial attempts I think they'll be worth it in the wear and tear they'll save on your nerves.

You see, it's really rather simple. With the above dinner, you'll want a dry white wine, and don't be deluded into thinking that the more expensive a wine, the better. There are numerous domestic wines, ranging in price from $.79 a bottle to $2.98 that are quite excellent. Buena Vista or Italian Swiss Colony are both acceptable. Santo Tomas and Paul Masson, superb.

Also you'll want lots of coffee, and not the instant kind. Some men don't object to instant coffee, but the majority do. Play it safe and brew it fresh.

If you've been managing your budget as well as I hope, you might be able to splurge on an after dinner something-or-other. Fine, there's nothing that does more to set off a good dinner, and put a man in a splendid state of comfort, than a good liqueur. Don't get too carried away in your choice, however. Many people just do not like porcupine quill brandy. Stick to something good, even though it's expensive. A small bottle of Courvoisier, Drambuie, or B and B, will pay off in handsome dividends and, reserved for special occasions when he's there, will last quite a long time.

Chances are that among your friends are some who are good or even excellent cooks. Now I may as well warn you, some of them will guard their recipes religiously. Frankly, I'm suspicious when a cook doesn't want to confess what is in a dish I'm eating. Be that as it may, the real chef will be flattered when you ask for a recipe, or a little coaching. Take advantage of his knowledge. The next time he invites you for dinner, ask if you can come early and help. Along with helping, you'll watch every move that he makes, and ask questions when you're puzzled. The next day, give him a call and ask if he'll write down the recipe for you, in plain language.

Putting out a good meal from time to time is not as difficult as non-cookers tend to think. In addition to using some of the short cuts such as already prepared foods, you can also save yourself a great deal of confusion if you'll do much of the preparation in advance. For the above dinner, as an example, the Jell-O salad can be made the night before. The onion can be chopped hours ahead of time, the margarine set out to melt, the bread cubes waiting in a bowl to be tossed. Shortly before he's due to arrive, you can make the coffee, and even put the corn into a saucepan, so all you have to do with it is turn on the fire.

There are also certain dishes that you'd best not attempt at first. It was years before I mastered Baked Alaska, and I have yet to fix a decent mousse (which is a dessert, and not a rodent). You're better off serving a plain steak which is good than an oyster soufflé which sounds more elegant, but turns out ghastly.

So much for the dinner itself. Now let's backtrack a little. There's more than food involved in making the evening successful and let's go into some of those details at this time.

Needless to say, you've cleaned the apartment thoroughly, preferably the day before so that you're not exhausted by the time he arrives. If the pace has been hectic, and you really are a little weary, try this: Lie down across the bed (before he comes, of course), with your head over the edge, and lower than your feet. Just relax like that for fifteen minutes, without falling asleep. It will do wonders for restoring your lagging energies.

Aside from the apartment, you yourself are clean and looking your loveliest. Even though you're at home, you're still working. You'll be wearing your new perfume, and just before he gets there, you might want to sprinkle a little of it around the apartment, just for reinforcement.

You'll use those old standbys, candlelight and soft romantic music. And the cocktail glasses will be in the refrigerator when he arrives, crisply chilled—that is, the glasses will be chilled, not him. If he is, offer to thaw him out.

Just in case you don't know how to make a cocktail, I'll provide the basics here. Your best bets will be martinis and Manhattans—there are few drinkers who won't consume one of the two.

In the case of a martini, I recommend vodka because it's cheaper than gin—unless he has expressed a preference for gin. Put some ice in a pitcher for mixing. The weakest you can get away with is four parts of vodka to one part of vermouth...a real martini drinker may want it even stronger. And, before you get confused, you're using the dry, white vermouth. Add a dash of olive juice from the jar, and drop an olive into the cocktail glass. Stir and serve.

As for a Manhattan, you'll substitute sweet (dark) vermouth for the dry, bourbon for the vodka. In this case, you can use a three-to-one mixture—Manhattan drinkers are a different breed. And for the olive, you'll substitute a cherry.

Those two recipes will see you through most dinners and cocktail events. But before I finish with the subject of drinks, I'll offer two more suggestions.

The Mollie Hogan is an ideal punch type drink for large gatherings when you don't want to go to the expense and work of cocktails. It's fine for holiday get-togethers. For this you'll need the juice of a dozen oranges, and the juice of 2 lemons, 6 teaspoons of vanilla, and ½ dozen eggs. Mix all of this thoroughly in an electric blender, or with an egg beater. Add 1 fifth of gin. Put some ice in a glass, pour 1 and ½ jiggers of the above mixture over it, and fill the glass with 7-Up. This should keep about 10 to 12 people in high spirits for a while.

The last drink recipe could also be used for a group, but the drinks have to be individually prepared, so it's a lot of work. Personally I think it's best saved for those evenings at home with him, preferably when the wind is howling outside and the fire and your emotions are keeping you cozy inside. Nothing can contribute more to your atmosphere of coziness than a toddy.

For this, you should have a big mug, or at least a large coffee cup. Hot toddies can be served in a glass, but they're a little hard to hold on to. Heat some water to boiling. Meanwhile, put in each mug a jigger or so of bourbon (this can also be done with Scotch, Irish, or rye whiskey). Add about 1 and ½ teaspoons of sugar, and a piece of stick cinnamon. Cut a lemon into wedges. Stick some whole cloves, about 3 or 4, into the lemon wedge (one garnished wedge for each cup), and drop that into the cup with the whiskey, etc. Finally, fill up the cup with boiling water, and serve. It will take a few minutes for the drink to cool down sufficiently to consume, but during this time it's soaking up all the spicy flavors. Incidentally, the stick cinnamon and whole cloves come from the spice rack at your market. As a bonus, this is a fine cure for general depression, or colds.

All right, that's it for your evenings with him. Remember to hide the dishes—a folding screen that blocks the kitchen off from view will save him the discomfort of glancing from the lovely table to that disaster area you've left in your wake. And never jump up from the table and start cleaning up the kitchen. He'll be obligated to help, and be in a far less romantic mood by the time you retire to the living room again. Half of your success depends upon creating and sustaining a mood of enchantment. Dirty dishes are not enchanting.

# CHAPTER EIGHT
## FRIENDS AND LOVERS

AS LONG as we're on the subject of entertaining, we may as well go into it more thoroughly. Some of your entertaining efforts may not be directly concerned with pursuing the Male Beast. Remember, though, I said directly. If you're really thinking right on the subject, virtually everything you do will be aimed at the same goal.

To illustrate—a little later I'm going to tell you all about stalking the brute, and some of my suggestions are going to rely upon friends, their parties, their acquaintances, etc. Now, as I said earlier, if you attend their parties and never extend them an invitation of any sort, you may suddenly find yourself off a lot of guest lists. Therefore, you have to entertain, even when there's no one in your group of guests that you're interested in.

Additionally, any entertaining you do gives you practice, so when you throw that party for a special one, you're an accomplished host. And even if you only have a few sisters in for coffee and cake, you have an opportunity to talk with them about their methods and accomplishments—special recipes they use, for instance, where they get their hair styled so nicely, what colors they think are best on you, and such. In any event, by now you like people, so you'll want to entertain some of them without furthering any ulterior motives.

Dinner for more than two will be much like the dinners you prepared in the last chapter, except that you'll add to the quantities I suggested. I may as well warn you, until you've acquired some real experience at preparing dinners, handling an affair of this sort for a dozen or more can be a nightmare. Best limit yourself to small dinner parties, of four or six people.

Your guests will sometimes offer to bring something. I don't generally approve of this, it somehow makes you seem less triumphant when things turn out well. However, you may want to let one of them bring the wine, and be sure to specify whether it should be red or white. An exception to doing it all yourself, by the way, would be a holiday type get-together of good friends, where everyone is supplying a dish, and the point is merely getting together to enjoy the holiday or special occasion.

Some people think nothing of inviting groups of people in and then parking them around on the floor with dishes, cups and saucers, napkins and eating utensils balanced on their knee caps. Frankly, I find this rather unsexy. A New Year's Day brunch, or a spur of the moment meal, or an outdoor barbecue if the facilities are available, might lend itself to this sort of serving. For the most part, however, a sit-down dinner will be much more impressive and enjoyable. I would rather use a board to increase the size of a table, and sit people on kitchen stools, than see them sprawled all about the apartment.

So much for dinners. Now we come to a very important type of entertaining—the cocktail party. They can be hellish to manage, but they can also be grand fun. A good host will be able to enjoy his party just as much as any of the guests. And notwithstanding the points I made at the beginning of the chapter, they can be very productive if you invite a few males you don't know well but want to become friendlier with, or if you suggest that your guests bring others—but make it a point to suggest that they bring a friend, or at least warn you of how many are coming, so you can be prepared.

I find it easiest to go for one of two extremes—a very small group, or a very large one. A group of twenty people find it difficult to share one conversation, nor is there that "room-full-of-people-to-mingle-with" atmosphere that lets a large party run itself.

For a small gathering, a dozen or less, you should look for common interests, or plan for the fact that all of your guests must be able to share the conversation and the fun. A group of this size is fine for party games or such, and if you're relying on conversations, it's up to you to keep them going, and see that everyone takes part.

Frankly I find a very large party easier. It calls for

more advance work and time, but once it gets going, it will generally sustain itself. In this case, follow a few rules:

Never have places for everyone to sit. Your early guests will tend to start forming circles—break them up. Keep your guests standing, and as a result, they'll circulate. This keeps a party moving, literally and figuratively.

Invite a genuine crowd—estimate how many people the room will hold, with chairs hidden away in closets, and add half a dozen or so to that number. Remember, not all of the invited guests will show up.

In either type party, try to stick to martinis and/or Manhattans. Invariably, you'll have the guest who asks for something else. Your answer will be that you don't have it. Not only does that make your party twice as expensive, but it means that you'll spend all your time mixing drinks to order, when, if you held to your resolution, they'd undoubtedly drink what you're serving. They'll get just as high and, even if they grumble, manage to have just as much fun...maybe more, because you'll be freer to see that they enjoy themselves.

My own method of serving drinks is an easy one, if you can find the right size bowls. I have a very large bowl which I fill with ice. Then I prepare my cocktails in a smaller bowl, which I then set on the ice. With a ladle, my guests are able to serve themselves just as they would at a punch bowl. The drinks stay cold, without being diluted, as they would if you just floated ice in the cocktails.

If you can't find bowls to work (I got mine in a dime store in clear glass for less than $1.00 each), get clear glass pitchers. Fill a bowl with ice water and set the pitchers into it. Don't fill the bowl with ice, as you'll spill the pitchers every time you replace them, and remember that they'll drip while pouring.

You'll need cocktail glasses. Regardless of what anyone tells you (and chances are it will be someone who gives dreadful parties), martinis do not taste the same in tea cups. Most cities have party supply houses from which you can rent cocktail glasses. They needn't be the finest crystal, but they do need to be stemmed.

It's the first half an hour that will make or break your party. During this time you must get your guests, those few who will arrive on time, to relax and start enjoying themselves. Give the very first ones something to do, such as setting up the drinks. Introduce the early arrivals to one another, but once the room starts filling up, drop this. By this time your guests will be meeting one another, starting conversations, and even flirtations. Every time you bring things to a halt to introduce a newcomer all the way around, it will be harder to get things going again. Introduce the newcomer to one group, or a particular person that you think he'll be interested in for one reason or another.

It will help if you have a friend or two whom you know are mixers and good conversationalists. In this case, steer the newcomer to this guest, particularly if the newcomer is the shy type, or a stranger to most of the people.

I've been to parties that were going along just beautifully, until the host came up with entertainment. The party itself should be entertainment. You'll need music when it starts, but by the time it really gets going, even that probably won't be needed. When you ask someone, who may be a lovely pianist or singer, to entertain, you risk boring those who aren't interested in classical music or show times. Such entertainment is fine for a small group, or when everyone has been invited for just that reason. Likewise, there are occasions that are ideally suited to group fun, such as Christmas Eve when probably everyone will want to sing carols.

There's one additional question that has to be covered, the question of whether a party should be gay, straight, or mixed. Obviously there will be times when an all gay party, or an all straight one, will be necessary. If it's the group from your office, it will probably be straight, and if it's just for your sisters, it will be gay.

While many homosexuals steer away from the mixed party, I personally find this type the most fun, and usually the most successful. For one thing, you can risk inviting the borderline male, the one you aren't sure about, and by the time the evening's over, you may be more knowledgeable.

Of course, it goes without saying that you'll warn your gay friends that it's mixed. Unless your friends are a pretty dreary sort, most of them will be on their good behavior. Of course, there will be the queen who gets a little high, and a little obvious, but if you warn the straight guests that some of your friends are a little kooky, they probably will take it in stride. At my last cocktail party, I had one guest who insisted on kissing, or trying to kiss, every man in the place good-bye. The gay friends thought it was funny, and the straight ones laughed too, but they understood that the fellow was just a little too drunk to know what he was doing. No one went home mortified or in a snit.

What else happened at that party? Well, that gorgeous creature whom I had wondered about but regarded as just "too" straight, ended up leaving, quite discreetly, with a sister. I later learned that this one wasn't too straight after all. I didn't get him, but my sister was happy over it all, and I moved this man's name to the "available" list. Next time, I'll know how to operate on him.

# CHAPTER NINE
## ALL ABOUT MEN

AT LAST, long last, we've come to the subject closest to our hearts—man. Actually, we've been on that subject all along, but now we have you prepared for the hunt, and we're ready to go.

Hunting a man is not much different from hunting any other wild animal, except that I think men are the wildest. We've already provided you with the proper weapons and other equipment, of course. But any good hunter will tell you that, in order to corner and capture your prey, you must first study the object of your pursuit. So let's look at our prey scientifically, all right?

There are three areas of knowledge that are necessary for making the kill. First, you have to know what a man is. Can you imagine going out after a tiger, without the vaguest idea what a tiger is? Second, you need to know everything possible about the animal's nature—his weaknesses, his strengths, his peculiarities. Third, there's the question of how we go about making the capture.

I can just hear you dismissing the first category

already. Everyone knows what a man is, you're saying. He's that beautiful tower of flesh with maddening eyes, with arms, legs, and other attachments.

If there is any single way in which gay fellows fail in the hunt, it's in not spotting their prey. Oh, they're aware of the male gender of those around them, but for some reason they insist on shooting some tigers and leaving the others free to romp about unmolested. This one isn't available, they say, or that one wouldn't be interested in me, and other such excuses. Sheer nonsense.

To my way of thinking, all men are Availables until they prove otherwise, and few of them have proved otherwise. Of course, there is a difference between desirable and undesirable Availables. I'm fully aware that Alcoholics Anonymous has helped many men to overcome their drinking problem, but it's not a task that I would particularly want to undertake myself. That applies also to drug addicts, psychopathic murderers, and other types of weirdoes.

But that leaves us with vast numbers of desirables, who are also Availables. Picture this scene, if you will: You are out with your sister, shopping, when you spot a perfectly adorable male creature. Both of you are tripping over your tongues as you follow him about. Then, when you've finally gotten close, you spy the ring on his finger. "Forget it," you tell your companion, "he's married."

It's a familiar scene, one that I've seen enacted numerous times. But if you're one of those who labors under the delusion that a man is no longer an Available because he's sporting a wedding ring, it's time you shed your leopard skin and moved into the twentieth century. I'll go into the types of men later, but for the present let's accept the fact that this adorable creature is a man. For the present, we'll assume that he's neither alcoholic nor drug addicted, nor anything of that sort. Therefore, he's available. He's fair game. Now that doesn't mean you'll get him—the hunter can't catch every tiger he spots either—but you can try.

A few years ago, I worked in an office with as attractive a young man as I've seen before or since. Not only was he attractive, but he was a thoroughly charming and likable sort. We became "office friends," and even associated out of the office. All the while, I chewed my nails in frustration and refrained from making a pass, fearful of the refusal I was certain I would get, and the consequences. So I suffered silent agonies when he put his arm around my shoulder or tickled me, and tried not to look into his eyes too closely.

When he stayed overnight at my apartment, I put him on the sofa and, after a hungry glance in his direction as he undressed in front of me, I scurried away to my bedroom. Once he phoned me in the middle of the night, getting me out of bed, and insisted that he had to see me right then to talk about something that was bothering him. I put him off.

Not until two years later, long after I had left that office, did I find out the truth. He was crazy about me, and even more frustrated than I was. And that middle of the night phone call was his attempt to bring matters to a head. At that moment, he was prepared to come to my apartment and take me by force if necessary—which wouldn't have been necessary at all.

By the next day, thinking that he had been tactfully refused, he offered an apology for the call, and a weak excuse. And by the time I learned all this, he was settled down with someone else. Once a month since then, without fail, I persuade one of my friends to kick me, just to remind me of how foolish I was.

It was a lesson that I never forgot, either. On another occasion I was with friends in a rather posh gay club. In walked a young man so stunning that all eyes in the place fell on him and stayed there. Everyone in the room was lusting after him as he seated himself alone at the bar and ordered a drink.

My friends, too, were flipping. "Why don't you go over and talk to him?" I suggested to one of them.

"You're kidding," was the reply. "He's too beautiful to be interested in anyone in this place."

Looking around the room, it suddenly occurred to me that everyone else there was thinking just the same thing. And after ten minutes, Mr. Beautiful was still sitting by himself.

"All right," I announced to my hesitant companion, who was certainly better looking than I. "If you don't want it, I'll take it."

With that, I marched to the bar and introduced myself to the young man. He was so friendly that it was quick to see that he was just plain lonely. Later, he told me that people rarely approached him in bars, because they thought he was unattainable. He wasn't, I can assure you. There was no hesitation on his part when I asked him to join our group, or later when I asked...but let's not go into details, I think you get the point.

Unless by some twist of Fate you are the sole male inmate of a woman's prison, you are surrounded by men. I'll admit some of them are stretching the point, but if nothing else they're good for practice. In the chapter on cruising, I mentioned the cop giving you the ticket, the insurance man, and others. All through the day, every day, there are countless men whose paths are crossing yours. It's up to you to trip a few of them.

There are men in your office, for one thing. If there aren't, it's time you took the man-hunter's pledge, or turned in your merit badges. Repeat after me: On my honor I will do my best to find, chase and capture men (substitute The Man if you're so inclined). Until I have achieved my goals, I will think men, work men, sleep men, eat and drink men (we're speaking symbolically), talk men, and collect men. Ah-men.

What about your relatives? I'm not proposing incest, although I've known some pretty close relatives who have kept it in the family, so to speak. But it gives you someone on whom to practice your wiles. If you've learned to use your baby blues to weaken Uncle Joe's resistance to your ideas, you can use them to convince the next available, too.

There's your clergyman, and your doctor, and your

dentist. There's the man at the supermarket, and the one at the service station. There are elevator operators, coffee counter busboys, cab drivers, door-to-door salesmen, your boss, the neighbor, the bartender at your favorite haunt, and the shoeshine boy at the corner. Look around you. If you don't know a man when you see one, all the rest of this is just wasted on you.

All right, now that we've established the basic identity of the brute, let's go into more detail. The more you know about the nature of man, the better your chances of success will be. Not all men are alike, so we'll start by examining the various sub-species.

ROMEO—everyone knows at least one Romeo. He's the Don Juan, the flirter, the love-them-and-leave-them conqueror of countless hearts. His efforts may be directed exclusively at women, or at men, or at either and both.

Romeo is an artist when it comes to love, romance, and sex. You'll learn more in one night with Romeo than I could teach you in twenty volumes. You owe it to yourself to have one fling with a Romeo. It will teach you a lot, and prepare you for the next Romeo, who might be the dangerous one for you. Besides, they are charming, exciting people who'll make you feel more beautiful and desirable than you've ever felt before.

My last encounter with a Romeo, two of them actually, was in Athens. The Greeks are a race of Romeos. My friend and I were literally picked off the streets by two of those famous Greek gods. Of course, we knew they had ulterior motives, very mercenary ones, but

I've never been hustled in more style.

They bought us drinks and toasted us as a welcome to Athens. They took us to dinner—not a noisy, tourist place, but an intimate little place on a rooftop. We could see the Acropolis in the distant moonlight. The musicians were called to our table and serenaded us. And we were fairly drowned in sweet nothings and enchanting compliments.

That's a Romeo. He is not marrying material unless you don't mind staying alone nights, or watching while he works on his latest conquest. What's more, he is not the one to fall in love with, hard as that may be. And when you do, which of course you will if he's set his mind to it, it will take a long time to get over him.

MR. MARRIED—I've mentioned this one before, and I've already pointed out that his married status does not make him unavailable, whether he's gay-married, or straight-married. What I didn't tell you was that he's a wonderful lover.

Why is he available, and a good lover? Well, depending upon how long he's been married, he's probably a little bored with what he's getting, regardless of the fact that he's in love with his mate. If you study primitive cultures, you'll find that while almost all of them sanctify marriage as an institution, almost all of them also make allowances for a certain amount of extra-marital activity.

That's because it's the nature of man to stray. Likewise, in our society, his chances to stray are somewhat limited. As a result, he's likely to take advantage of whatever opportunity presents itself, which means you. As a bonus, he's already had some training in being thoughtful and agreeable, and some experience in bedroom techniques.

Married men often tend to be more generous. I suppose it's their way of compensating for the limitations they have to put on the affair. Likewise, you won't have to share him with any of your friends.

Like Romeo, Mr. Married is not the one to get too involved with. There's always the outside chance that he'll leave his wife and family for you, but better not count on it. If you do fall in love with him, there's only one cure. Go look for another Romeo.

THE BRAIN—as a category, the Brain is hard to describe accurately. If you can get the mind stopped long enough to put the body in motion, you may find yourself with a tornado. Some of them, however, never get that far, and there's no way to tell without trying.

On the other hand, they can certainly be interesting and stimulating, and they are often available for settling down. If they decide on you, they usually won't bother flirting with anyone else, and you'll only have to share them with their lofty thoughts.

THE ATHLETE—I've included the body beautiful in this category, the genuine athlete, and even the enthusiast-to-the-core, so it's a varied group, but there are sufficient similarities that mark the breed.

Except for the armchair enthusiast, and then not always, they are usually dull as lovers. In fact, they're often dull out of bed as well. There's a good chance that the Athlete will never love anyone because his heart belongs to himself.

So why bother at all? Well, there's one thing in their favor, they are usually attainable. They are devoted to the male ideal, and while they may go through the motions with a female, it's the male body that really gets to them. The professionals and body builders are also terribly accustomed to male companionship and body contact. I recently read an article about professional football players. The wives of these men lead a lonely life, because they have to take second place to the men in their husband's lives. These men travel together constantly, sharing rooms, showers, beds, meals, and everything else. Obviously, they can't be too opposed to the male sex.

What's more, this category is much like a lovely piece of jewelry—not very practical, but lovely to wear and display. Don't be afraid to wear one occasionally, even if they do become boring quickly.

TOP BRASS—the business executive, or Top Brass, is pure gold. Consider the facts: he obviously has quite a bit on the ball to have gotten where he is. He has polish, a sense of responsibility, self-confidence, etc.

Of course, he's also hard to get. You usually can't fool him as to the worth of anything. You'll have to be worth his interest, but you've got something in your favor there, too—he's accustomed to looking below the surface, for the real value. Looks are less important than charm, breeding, wit, and other merits.

Discretion is a must with the executive—his entire career, which is probably his life, is at stake. Once he's assured of this discretion on your part, however, he'll be slower to change partners than some other types.

Flexibility is another asset you'll need. His mood may be serious and concerned with the office, and all of your efforts will be wasted on him. Another time he'll forget the office and be yours exclusively, so be patient. If he's promised to arrive no later than seven, and his boss keeps him late, don't complain. By keeping his boss happy, he can better afford those nice gifts for you.

THE ARTIST—this one is probably the easiest to get into bed, which in my opinion makes him the least rewarding. Taken with care, they can be fun and entertaining, and certainly stimulating. This is your opportunity to wear those way-out clothes and be the madcap you've sometimes dreamed of being. Don't make it a habit, though, it tends to scare away other, more desirable types. And not too madcap, either. That cigarette that tastes so peculiar may be your invitation to all sorts of problems.

THE COLLEGE BOY—with things being what they are today, the College Boy is generally pretty much available. It's become an IN thing at big universities and colleges to dabble in a few lavender pastimes, and he doesn't want to seem square. If he hesitates, display a few Jean Genet books around—chances are good he's a Genet fan, like most College Boys, and Genet will help you convince him that boys can be fun.

The College Boy will combine some of the elements of the Brain and the Athlete, because he'll probably be interested in both mental and physical activities. He's also fun and interesting, if a bit boorish at times. Don't expect him to be too good in bed—he hasn't had the experience yet to be an artist—but he may make up for that in youthful energy, fresh young skin, and other attributes of youth.

THE YOUNGSTER—this is a touchy subject, needless to say, but I'm not advocating that you should whisk little Junior from next door off to your boudoir. If you've already got a thing for the Youngsters, nothing I can say is going to change your tastes.

What I am advocating, however, is that you take advantage of legitimate opportunities to learn and benefit from these young devils. You may have a job, such as teaching, that keeps you in contact with them, and if not there are undoubtedly certain occasions when you are around them, if only briefly.

Young men, whether homosexually inclined or not, are instinctive and superb flirts, far better at it than they will be later, in adulthood. At this point in their lives, flirting, by one name or another, is the only way they've had of getting attention and their way in things. I have a nephew who isn't old enough to know what this puberty things he's in means, and he knows more about the art of flirting than I'll ever be able to remember.

There's no better cure for feeling unsexy than to be around a young man for even a few minutes. He could put any Romeo to shame, and teach you just as much, or more.

Some of them, I must admit, are available—in fact, some of them are more determinedly on the prowl than you'll ever be. But I think it only fair to warn you, no matter what he does to seduce you, and they are seducers, no matter if he overpowers you physically and forces you to submit to his desires—when you get caught, he is innocent and you are guilty.

I'm not criticizing you for your idea of fun, I'm just warning you not to cry on my shoulder.

G.I. JOE—the military man is like the College Boy in many respects, including his probable age. Likewise, he's generally available. Like the Athlete, he's accustomed to male companionship and body contact, maybe even more so. In history, and even today in societies other than ours, homosexuality is taken for granted among these fighting men. Even in our military society, homosexuality is pretty common.

The military man has a masculine image to maintain, and he's taking a lot of risk in addition. That means that what he'll do alone with you and what he would admit to around his buddies or want his buddies to suspect are two different things entirely.

Strangely enough, the Marine Corps, while enjoying a reputation as being the butchest of the services, is also the one regarded as the "gayest," at least so far as being available. They're also the roughest, and most dangerous, if that bothers you.

Next best bet, I'm told, is the Navy. Even more so than the other branches of service, Navy men are alone together for long periods of time. It's a rare sailor who absolutely opposes an occasional homosexual encounter.

The Army also offers some good possibilities, while the Air Force generally seems to provide the poorest selection of Availables.

THE PROTECTORS—I've put the rest of the uniformed men in this category—the policeman, fireman, etc. Statistics tell us that the highest percentage of men with homosexual leanings are to be found in these professions, probably because of the association of masculinity with the appeal of the uniform. Be that as it may, I have a friend who swears by firehouses. It's difficult, he tells me, to become accepted among the men, but once you're in, anything (and everyone) goes.

As for policemen—let's be honest, your chances are slim. Not because they don't lean that way, which they do, but because they have to be so careful. I have another friend who just dotes on uniformed policemen, and has had an impressive number of successful encounters. On the other hand, he's also had a few arrests, which is a risk of the game.

If you feel that your trophy room just won't be completed until you've added a policeman, be sure to go slow, make your hints as ambiguous as possible, and be careful to offer him a maximum of privacy and discretion.

THE VIRGIN—sooner or later you're going to run into the perpetual virgin. He will flirt, lead you on, pat you as you pass, and in general drive you to distraction—only to announce, when you attempt to take him up on all those offers, that he doesn't do that sort of thing. Ignore him, and remember that the laws regarding murder are quite strict.

MR. ORDINARY—if you're planning on a long-term investment, Mr. Ordinary is the man you want He's almost impossible to define as a category, because Mr. Ordinary may come from the upper, middle, or lower classes. He may drive a taxi, sell neckties in a department store, or work as a bookkeeper in a dingy office somewhere. He's rarely breathtakingly lovely, although often nice-looking, rather unexciting out of bed and often positively mad between the sheets, pleasant to be around in a comfortable fashion, and altogether quite human.

Be comfortable with Mr. Ordinary, make him comfortable too, and learn to relax and be yourself.

It goes without saying that a list of this sort could go on and on, but I think the above categories will give you plenty to work on as a start.

* * * * * * *

Before going on to the pursuit of our prey, however, let's conclude our study of his nature by covering some elementary facts that are common to most men. There are five things that men like. In order of usual preference, they are:

1.) themselves—it's called male ego, and it's universally common in one degree or another. More important, he wants you to share his good judgment. He will overlook your walk, the way you talk, or the limp condition of your wrist, before he'll risk losing your respect, admiration, and, most of all, the attention you shower on him.

2.) sex—this is the ace in the hole for our side. Those who grew up on the farm have probably tried it with all sorts of animals. The city bred have tried it with one another, or the neighborhood kids, or whatever was available. There's no reason why he can't be persuaded to try another variation on the theme.

3.) companionship—this one might very well have gone before sex, but I thought it was more accurate this way. Ideally, the man likes these two combined, but he's not above getting them separately. Fortunately, you can combine them. One thing is certain, however, regardless of how much sex he's getting, and enjoying, he will still want and need companionship. Sell him on yours, and then work on sex.

4.) men—no, I'm not saying all men are homosexual, in the usual sense of the word. But according to history, psychology, sexology, and every other ology, men do prefer the company of men. Put him in the company of a group of women, and the more heterosexual a man is, the more uncomfortable he will be. He enjoys bedding women. Out of bed, he prefers the boys.

5.) being men—this is close to the same thing as liking themselves, but they like to think of themselves, and be thought of, as men. And we like them to be the same. So never stop telling him and implying in every possible way that he is all man. Once you start calling him Miss, or referring to him as your wife, you're defeating his male image, and maybe driving him into the arms of someone else with whom he can be a man.

Sound simple? It is, actually. As I told you in the very beginning, it's mostly a matter of common sense. Of course, I'm only offering some very simplified notes. Man can also be a terribly complicated subject, but then, I suppose that's one of the things that makes him so attractive.

# CHAPTER TEN
## HAUNTS AND HABITS

FINDING a man is just like finding any other animal one happens to be hunting—you have to go where they are. In the case of men, this is relatively easy, because they are in so many places. However, not all of those places lend themselves as well to your kind of hunting. Too, the locale of your search will depend upon the type you're looking for, and your ultimate goals.

If, for instance, sex is your only motivation, a steam bath will probably provide the answer. If you're looking for something more serious than that, you should look elsewhere.

The bar is the most obvious hunting grounds, particularly the gay bar. Mind you, I did not say it was the most desirable or satisfactory. It's true, you'll have a variety to choose from and work on. On the other hand, you'll have more competition.

Likewise, in a gay bar, you run the risk of hustlers, vice officers, and other such disappointments. It's also said that your chances of a long-lasting relationship are slimmer, but I can't really say that I agree. I've known some fairly long-term affairs that began with bar pickups. In the long run, the durability will depend upon you and your makeup, and to a lesser degree upon his (part of your job is convincing him, so his views are less important on this subject).

Many homosexuals have a tendency to limit themselves by going to gay bars exclusively. This, in my estimation, is unfortunate, and deprives them of some perfectly wonderful opportunities. Oh, yes, cruising does go on in that swanky hotel bar, whether you're in Beverly Hills, or Indianapolis. It's more discreet, of course, but by now you've mastered that art. There's a bonus, too—the swank spots are less plagued by vice officers and hustlers.

You may run into that out-of-town salesman whose work is finished for the day and who, miles from home and friends, is quite lonely for someone to talk to. Speaking as one who has worked with them, salesmen are actually a very lonely group, and they are frequently quite broadminded. And if not a salesman, you may meet the visiting executive. I spent an evening with one of Broadway's most illustrious producers, merely because he was on the West Coast on business, and lonely when I happened by. Needless to say, the meeting took place on Beverly Hills' plush Wilshire Boulevard, not in a back alley bar.

Perhaps the best method of meeting men is through your friends, gay and straight. You'll meet some without any real prompting on your part. Never turn down invitations to parties and such, without a really valid reason. Even the dullest party may produce golden opportunities. What's more, at a party it's easy to get things started. Obviously you have mutual acquaintances and interests, so there's groundwork for conversation, and if you drift over to a man and strike up a conversation, you'll be regarded as a good party mixer, not a prowling pervert. And one of you may need a ride home.

Those talents that earn you invitations, for obvious reasons, are valuable. Bridge can be learned with a little effort, and bridge players are always looking for a fourth. If you can play the piano, you might want to offer your services for entertainment at a party, but see to it you do some playing away from the piano.

One friend insists that he never had so much fun at a party as he did the New Year's Eve he offered to be bartender. He met literally everyone at the party, and was on extremely friendly terms with many of them by the time the party was over.

Anything that you can do to broaden your interests and put yourself in contact with more people will help. You might consider additional schooling. Almost every city has some sort of adult classes available in the evening, and you're certain to become friendly with some of your classmates, maybe even the teacher. And like the party, you have several advantages in this case—mutual interests, for one thing.

Your job is another important area, but it's so important that I'm saving that for a separate chapter.

Join up with a local opera company (they always need people to carry spears) or theater group. Whatever your interests are, from stamp collecting to horseback riding, there are others nearby who share them. Join in—you'll not only improve yourself, but you'll have fun, and meet new people—maybe the right one.

Sports is another subject of interest. Now I know you may not be able to make a basket without weaving, and balls just don't sound to me like something I want to hit with a stick. Frankly, I'm remembered by one startled host as the person who thought Sandy Koufax was a rock and roll singer. (I'm still not sure just what he does have to do with football.)

But sports mean men. I thought that would make your ears perk up. At the very least, you can be a watcher, and you may find eventually that you want to try your hand at something or other. In every sport, there are people who aren't very good, but they play anyway, and enjoy themselves, and meet all sorts of men.

For instance, I can't imagine anything duller than a game like golf, but every time I pass a course and see all of those lovely men wandering around, I reconsider. It might be the one game you'd be really good at.

There's tennis, which is certainly chic, and healthy. You can wander over to the courts by yourself and hit at the ball for a while. Don't be surprised if you soon have a partner. Even if you don't want to be that active, no one questions a bystander at a tennis court, where you can stand all afternoon and watch those naked masculine legs.

There's skiing, which seems a little dangerous to me,

besides getting out where it's cold. But it does mean you could wear those devastating outfits, and you can always stay in your room at the lodge until cocktail time.

Skating, either ice or roller, is also fine. And here again, you can stand and watch all evening without anyone getting suspicious. Of course, as in anything else, if you participate you have more likelihood of getting acquainted.

What if all of this is too active for you? Then you can still spend the afternoon at the beach, where there's plenty of fresh air, sunshine, and men in various stages of undress. Needless to say, you're not just going to sit there. Take along a radio, which can be tuned into the ball game (dull, but it attracts men), or a controversial book, or even a deck of cards. A game of solitaire might net you a partner for something else.

Let me remind you once more that you don't need a crowd around you. Most people would be a little scared away by an entire mob of fellows bunched together on the sand.

There are racetracks, which sometimes attract some interesting men. Of course, he may be too broke afterward to take you to dinner. There are also boxing and wrestling matches, but I can't imagine anyone being that desperate. If you live in California, of course, there's the roller derby. I've never gone, but I've heard that it can be quite productive for a queen.

Some areas have homosexual clubs and groups. I'm not very familiar with most of these, but you might want to investigate the possibilities.

Conventions can be interesting, depending upon the type. Political conventions, for instance, are generally not satisfactory. Other conventions, however, can be marvelous. Sales conventions, auto shows, and such, are well worth looking into. I've already mentioned that out-of-town salesmen can be a joy. Pretend you have lots of money to spend, and don't be shy.

Vacations are grand, depending upon where you go, with whom, and such. Most people tend to lose their inhibitions as they get away from home, for some peculiar reason. I'm always more brazen on foreign soil.

If you have friends in the town you're visiting, fine. If not, you may want to check out some of the gay spots, but don't forget the bar in your hotel, of course. As for finding the gay spots—cab drivers, particularly if they see a couple of dollars in your hand, usually know where to send you. Likewise with bartenders. Or you can follow the first swishy number you see on the street.

There are also guide books, but my own experience suggests that these aren't reliable. Look a place over for yourself before deciding that it's really gay, regardless of what the guidebook says.

Of course, you may want to plan your vacation to a particular location, or at a particular time, when you know things will be jumping. Mardi Gras, for instance, is legendary, and there are Mardi Gras in cities other than New Orleans.

There are also music and film festivals, some of

which are nice, some deadly. Summer opera seasons also seem to attract interesting men.

As for where—take your pick. Most cities offer some possibilities. New York, San Francisco, Los Angeles, and Chicago are most famous for the gay life, but again, remember that competition will be tougher.

There are all the western resorts, filled with handsome, masculine rangers. One thinks they would get lonely. Anyway, the sights are lovely.

There's always Europe; for the homosexual who can afford it, it can be quite an experience. But that will require another book, I'm afraid.

In addition to where and when, there's a question of how to travel. Time, and money, will have some bearing on this. Personally, if it's a long trip, I'd rather fly and have more time and money to spend there. And in fact, for one person, flying is not much more expensive than any other way of traveling, considering your free meals, etc.

Busses and trains can be interesting. I have never personally done anything on either, other than getting acquainted and laying some groundwork. I have friends, however, who have laid a great deal more, including fellow travelers. That would be one way to pass the time. And most people on these vehicles are bored, with a lot of time on their hands. Chances are that man, practically trapped in the seat next to you, will welcome your conversation.

The same is true of planes, except that they move faster, so you'll have to do likewise. And you certainly don't want an elderly lady, charming though she may be, occupying the seat next to you. Sneeze when she starts to sit down, or have a coughing fit. You have things to accomplish.

Traveling by car is, in my estimation, a bore. Long hours of staring at highways, and you never meet anyone. There are hitchhikers, of course, but some of the relationships that have sprung up from that start are to be found in newspaper headlines. The chances that you'll wind up a "victim" are always high.

I mentioned your neighbors before, and by now I hope you've taken some notice of them.

There's always shopping. If the store you patronize doesn't have any attractive clerks, shop at another store. Most of the merchandise is the same anyway, so you might as well look for other bonuses.

There's even church; I've met some very interesting people after the sermon.

So you see, they're to be found almost everywhere. Are you pulling into just any service station, when the one a few blocks down the street has gorgeous attendants? Shame on you.

Of course, there are places you shouldn't meet them, and ways, just as there are men who are undesirable. Blind dates may be awfully dull, unless arranged by a good friend, and mysterious voices on the phone can lead to trouble. So can public parks and restrooms, I'm sorry to say. The same goes for steam baths, and those streets that are notorious for pickups—Selma Avenue in Hollywood, and those others you're always hearing about.

No, the sailors do not stand in rows to be picked out on the main streets of San Diego, the fellows in the park in Washington do not have sexual intercourse on the ground in plain sight, Central Park is not Heaven, and most of the bare beaches are overrated. But you can try all those for yourself if you like, and if you like to live dangerously. It just seems silly to me, when you have all those other places to look.

# CHAPTER ELEVEN
## BRING 'EM BACK ALIVE

NOW the fun begins; your guns are properly loaded and you're on the prowl. From here on, you'll need to be constantly alert, all of your senses in high gear.

You've picked out your hunting grounds, and your prey. Ideally, you'll want to take time to study him, every move, every gesture. You'll identify his type, and look for his vulnerable spot. Of course, there are some times when you'll have to work fast. When you walk into the bar and see, just as you seat yourself, the one you want, who is plainly bored, and plainly preparing to leave, you may not have the time to attack scientifically. This is like the hunter who spots his prey on the run. Better to take a few wild shots, in the hope that one of them will catch him, than to let him escape unmolested. Several of the techniques I'm going to mention below will serve in this situation as well. Pick one of them, and try it. It might be just the one to slow his escape.

There are many possibilities for meeting men in bars, or elsewhere. For one thing, you can make a "partner in crime" of the bartender, by becoming a regular. Particularly if it's a gay bar, he will be helpful in steering you toward the safe customers, and away from the unsafe or unavailable. He may even be able to arrange introductions to some of the other regulars. Likewise, if you become a regular, you will certainly have become at least casually acquainted with some of the other customers, who might also be able to introduce you to that interesting newcomer. There is a difficulty in this; you will become familiar and thus less interesting to some of the patrons.

Most of the time, it will be up to you to get the ball rolling. This is where you need your wits about you, and if possible, the time to study your victim. Even the most trivial detail or action on his part may give you the clue you need in determining the best approach.

Without doubt the most universal approach is the old workhorse, the mistaken identity technique. It does sometimes work, but it has certain flaws also. If your victim interrupts you, for instance, to point out that you've made a mistake, you're out of business. The only way to counter this is to begin by flattering him. If you walk up from behind and say to him, "It has to be Jack Jiblets, there couldn't be two bodies that beautiful," you've managed to score points before he even looks at you.

The real weakness in this technique, however, is the fact that it is overused, and lacks imagination. If he has anything on the ball, he's hardly going to be impressed by your lack of originality. For this reason, I prefer to use the mistaken identity technique as an emergency measure, to be used when no other clue presents itself, or in those situations I mentioned previously where you have to do something fast before he gets away. Usually however, you'll be able to find a clue.

I can only offer a few examples of such clues, and how they are used to your advantage. The possibilities are endless, but once your own imagination starts working, you'll rapidly get the hang of it.

Jewelry is often an excellent way of starting the conversational ball rolling. Even if he proves to be not interested in you, he can't be offended when you compliment him on his ring or cuff links. If there's no jewelry to be seen, you can carry this a little further and comment on his suit, asking for the name of his tailor or haberdashery. If nothing else, his complexion may be the very opening you need. For instance, suppose it's midwinter where you are, and he's sporting a golden tan. In that case, you start with, "Excuse me, but I've been wondering where you got that beautiful tan in this weather." Be careful to say "tan" and not "brown" as in the mistaken identity technique, you are beginning this one by complimenting him, which automatically weakens his resistance.

It may be his conversation that provides the answer. If he asks the bartender the score of the game, you don't need to know what game to ask the same question of your prey. It's a small opening, but it's an opening. Likewise, his voice may tell you that he's not a native of the area—show him a little local hospitality.

Needless to say, once you've started the conversation, no matter how slightly, you have to keep it going. He may make this easy for you by responding at length, and incidentally revealing an area of interest to him which you can pursue. If, however, the conversation falters after the discussion of his cuff links, then you can try a change of direction. "Are you in the jewelry business?" or "Are you in town on business?" for example.

If his response to your efforts leaves you stricken with frostbite, I'm afraid you've struck out. Don't let it discourage you, look for another one. At least you've practiced starting conversations, and as you've gathered by now, I'm a firm believer in practice.

These same techniques can be used out of bars as well—at the theater, a party, even shopping. Timing is essential in all of them; you have more in mind than just passing away a few minutes in idle conversation. You must learn to judge when the conversation should be steered away from such generalities and into more specific channels. His reactions to you may help you judge the time for this; give him time to warm up to you and relax. Then move slowly and carefully— suggest, if he's an out-of-towner, that you show him around a little. In some situations, however, boldness will be more successful than caution. "I'm on my way to dinner, would you care to join me?" or "Why don't we drop by my apartment and have a drink there, where we can relax?" are direct and sometimes ideal approaches.

If you're going for the direct line, remember that

you'll just have to strike out some of the time. Don't let it discourage you; the more times you try, the better the averages in your favor will be.

If you're meeting him because you are both members of the neighborhood bridge club, or theater group, things are much easier. You already have a subject for conversation, but use it to your best advantage. Why not ask for his help or suggestions? He'll be flattered if you begin by telling him that you admire his card or stage technique, and ask for a few pointers.

There's an additional gimmick you can use effectively, that sometimes works perfectly. If you are fortunate enough to have a female friend who knows the score, and doesn't object to it, take her along with you to some of the bars, parties, and the like. For some peculiar reason, you can get away with a great deal more while you're holding her hand. Even if you make your interests obvious from the beginning, he'll still think of you as a man, rather than a faggot. Many men will not hesitate to have a little fun with a man, when they want nothing to do with faggots.

You won't always need introductions. This is the beauty of meeting them through friends, office, and such, where you are already acquainted and ready to move on to the question of bedding him.

Seduction is a science. And don't let that word frighten you. For centuries, men and women have been practicing it, sometimes in extremely devious and even diabolical forms. There's absolutely no reason why you shouldn't do the same.

I must warn you before we begin, however, that there is no room in seduction for fair play. You'll have to accept the philosophy that the end justifies the means—how badly do you want his end? Afterward, when he's yours, you can be as honest, as fair, as above reproach as you wish, but while you're working on him, you'll have to resign yourself to being a cad, it's that simple.

This is where we start using the information we've already gathered about men in general, not to mention what we've learned through careful observation and listening, about him in particular.

First, and foremost, appeal to his masculine self-image. Remember, he likes himself, and he likes to be a man. This does not mean that you have to become a sweet, helpless little thing terrified of anything so manly as opening a can of beans. It means that you act like a man, more or less, and always let him act like one. He is important, strong, wise, brave, generous, sensible, handsome, and just plain wonderful. You are not quite trivial, but certainly nowhere near as important as he is; definitely not weak, but far from possessing his strength; not helpless but in need of his protection and assistance; intelligent but without his profound wisdom; unbrave without being a constant scaredy-cat; not so much generous as giving him his due, which is everything; and you feel attractive with others, but when you're with him he makes you feel almost plain by comparison.

When you're out with him, find unobtrusive ways to slip him the money for your share and let him pay.

The first time or two you may feel a little awkward, but notice the way his chest swells slightly. That's progress, through his weakest spot, his ego.

If you'll do a little reading, you'll learn that many authorities are expressing concern over the respective roles of men and women in our society. Men, they insist, are being emasculated by women. She is hard at work to prove that he is no more important than she, and not at all superior. Once the man was called upon to defend her—now the chances are she may be better at karate than he. He was the breadwinner, the one qualified to deal with business and money. Now she earns more than he, and manages it better than he does, and tells him about it at every opportunity.

That's fine, because so long as his ego is suffering at her efforts, it's all the more susceptible to your efforts. As a matter of fact, Kinsey and others have pointed out that modern woman sometimes drives man into homosexual relationships. The divorced man who has gotten stung on alimony, or the single man who has just fought his way out of a breach of promise or paternity suit, may turn to a male lover for sexual outlet for the simple reason that it costs him less, financially and mentally. All of this, needless to say, is operating in your favor. From the standpoint of potential, I doubt if the homosexual has had it this good at any other time in history.

I've already mentioned being a good listener. This is the big key to being a successful conversationalist, but not the entire formula. Sooner or later he may wonder if you're a mute, or simply too stupid to say anything. Start conversations when necessary, and spur them along when they falter. Learn to feel him out on various subjects, until you learn which one interests him, and then pry the lid off his interest. Get him to express his opinion at length. Getting him to admit that Bette Davis is his favorite singer isn't enough; ask him why, and what are the songs she sings best.

The things that interest him are the things that interest you. When he says he likes the paintings of Winston Churchill, you are certainly not going to roll on the floor with laughter, tears streaming from your eyes as you scream, "You've got to be kidding!" He wasn't, and he's not going to believe that you were either when you apologize, if you ever get the chance. Likewise, if his interest in music goes no farther than "St. Louis Blues," he's only going to be bored listening to your description of the Metropolitan Opera opening.

I should point out a very important fact: being interested in his favorite subject does not necessarily mean being knowledgeable. You can pretend interest, you can't fake knowledge. If you try to convince him you know all about his subject, you may make your deception embarrassingly obvious, and convince him you're a fake. Everyone, of course, uses fakery from time to time, but it's like the genitalia, kept hidden in polite society.

As a matter of fact, ignorance will pay you far better dividends. This gives him a chance to show off his knowledge (since he can see you're interested) and build his ego a little. And it also gives you an opening for a future get-together. If opera is his specialty, and you sigh and say you've never seen one but it sounds like the most fascinating thing you've ever heard of, he just might invite you to the next one.

The same applies to sports, which as I said before is a favorite subject of many men. Encourage him to tell you all about football or baseball, and then say, "I'd love to see a game, and I can get tickets, but I don't like to go by myself. I need someone who could explain things to me."

Having started on companionship, your next task is to insure that he likes your company, and continues liking it. Never stop working to uncover his interests, all of them, his tastes, his special likes and dislikes. If he doesn't like flowers, paint over the cabbage roses in the dining room when you know he's coming. If he's a married man, gently encourage him to talk about his home life. In the course of the conversations, you'll learn what he thinks is wrong with his home life, the mistakes his wife (or lover) makes. Profit from them. If he likes boiled filet of motorcycle boot, which she won't prepare, you'll exclaim, "Heavens, I've been dying to fix some, but I don't know anyone else who likes it, and it's too much to fix for just one person." I'll bet my last boot he won't turn down a dinner invitation.

If his wife never listens to his problems after a bad day at the office, tape your ears so that they stand out prominently, and offer him all the sympathy he can take without suffering syrup poisoning. Next bad day, he'll head for you instead of home.

One word of warning—let him complain about his other half, and cluck sympathetically, but don't make the mistake of joining him in the attack. His sense of loyalty will necessitate his taking her side, and you're suddenly a common enemy.

Psychologically, we all enjoy doing things for others, which leaves them obligated to us, rather than have them doing things for us, which makes us feel obligated. A person will like you more if you ask him for something than if you shower him with gifts. Therefore, you want to make him feel important by asking him to give—of his company, because you're lonely and just can't face that apartment by yourself, for instance. If he enjoys cooking—many men do—ask him to prepare a meal or a dish. Make sure that you ask for something he enjoys doing, and nothing too extreme, of course. Even if he loves carpentry, he may not be enthusiastic about building an extra room on your house.

Thus far, you've been working on establishing a relationship of companionship between the two of you. Of course, you want it to go much farther. If he's gay, and you know it, things are simpler for you. If you're not sure, or even if you think he's not, you still stand a good chance.

All the while, you've been discreet about the relationship. Most important, you have given him nothing to apologize to others for—his buddies, the people at the office, or anyone. You haven't even broadcasted the friendship, although of course you aren't sneaking around about it either.

You've managed to take advantage of four of those five basic likes he has—himself, because you've shown you approve of and share his taste; companionship, which you've now established; men, which you've been acting like; and being a man, which you have encouraged him to be at all times. That leaves only one field of interest as yet untouched—sex. Now you're ready to start working on this.

Of course, maybe sex was all you were interested in, and it made little difference with whom, just anyone who is available. Fine, take the direct approach, shrug off those who say no and enjoy those who say yes.

This chapter is concerned with seduction, not just fornicating. I'm assuming this is someone who might, if asked cold, turn you down. You may also be looking for a more lasting relationship, rather than a one night stand. In either case, you need a campaign. And even if you're only looking for a one night stand, some of the best ones are the ones you have to work to get. But I'll leave it up to you. If you only want quick sex partners, and you have plenty of them available to you, fine. Otherwise, you'd better read on.

The first essential in successfully seducing him will be togetherness. This is, contrary to what you might think, something different from companionship. Think about it, you can be in someone's company and not really be together, right? This, then, is the crucial point that you must be able to cross.

In its most elementary terms, togetherness is a

matter of joining with him, making yourselves into a team. This is achieved in many subtle ways, some of them actually quite simple. For instance, if there is an argument in progress, put yourself on his side. He'll admire your good sense while condemning the others as idiots; what's more, you've established togetherness. You are the person who thinks as he does, who shares his feelings. In that state of mind, when it's firmly established, he'll be more likely to share your opinions—and desires.

If you're involved in team activities—games or such, you want to be on his team. Even if you don't do very well, he's still being saturated with togetherness. Of course, if you're really dreadful at whatever the game is, warn him firmly of this beforehand. If he insists, give it a try. Otherwise, remain on the sidelines, rooting for him—whatever you do, don't join with his opponents, even if you thus help them to lose. His victory, in that case, still won't offset your loss.

Join in whatever he does, as his teammate or, if he has a special activity, his companion. If he spends an hour each week working with the blind, go with him. If he's bartender at the party, get behind the bar and pitch in. After the dinner party suggest that you and he do the dishes while the others have their coffee.

If it's possible, take trips together. He may have to travel occasionally in his job, and he may welcome your company. Not only are you working on togetherness, but you're taking advantage of the fact that most people leave some of their inhibitions at home. He'll do far more in a hotel in Topeka than he will at home.

Once you've established togetherness between you, your next step is to take it from the psychological realm to the physical realm. Your first step in doing this will be body contact.

Now I'm not suggesting that you suddenly start pinching his fanny, or that sort of thing, except on rare occasions when you can get away with it as a joke. There will be those occasions, particularly if he's the sort to "horse around" with the other fellows. These occasions will require split-second timing on your part, if they're to be successful.

For instance, in a joking manner you sit on his lap. If this is not treated as a joke, it may cause him to withdraw from you. On the other hand, if it's treated entirely as a joke, it's wasted. The pose must be retained just beyond the joke stage, to that point where you suddenly discover that it's enjoyable and he finds himself inexplicably aroused by contact with your body. Not one second sooner or later, you must quickly end the contact, jumping up from his lap.

Your reaction should be slight embarrassment, while still trying to laugh it off. You don't want him to know or suspect that this was premeditated. You do, however, want to leave him with an unconscious desire for more.

There is a subconscious factor working in your favor, that will make him want more without being aware of the desire for what it is. It's called a conditioned reflex, but don't let that term frighten you. Basically, it is an established pattern of reaction to certain things. The

Russians began it by discovering that, if they rang a bell while feeding a dog, he learned to associate the bell with food. Eventually, whenever they rang the bell, he would display the same reactions as he did to food.

It's not really complicated—what you want to do is ring dem bells that are already built into him through his other experiences with sex. You see, in the past, even if his entire experience with sex has been with females, the feel of a fanny against his you-know-what meant sex. By now, without any conscious thought about it, his body is going to react the same way to that touch.

In other words, and to put it in the most elementary terms, that sort of touch, regardless of who's involved, will start off a sexual reaction in him. Now if you pushed it farther, his mind, the conscious part of it, would come into the act, and he'd have the chance to convince himself he doesn't go for that sort of thing. This is why it's necessary to stop at that point where his subconscious is working but his conscious hasn't caught on yet.

The conditioned reflexes he has learned in the past are an asset you'll use time and time again, in numerous ways. For instance, you'll learn to drop your arm about his shoulders, very lightly and very casually, as though you weren't even thinking about it. Preferably, you'll keep his conscious mind occupied with a conversation in which he's very interested. Without thinking of it, he may put his arm around you. This can be very easy to get away with if you're seeing him out, for instance.

Make it brief, and as a result he'll go out wanting more such contact. You see, if this were a girl, he would go further and kiss her good night. He won't, of course, but for a fleeting instant the desire is there. Each time this occurs, the desire will be a little stronger. By the time it filters through to his conscious mind, his resistance to it will already be quite weakened.

For this reason, you take advantage of body contact at every legitimate opportunity. In shaking hands, allow your hand to linger in his just a second or two longer than is necessary, covering up the move by thinking of something additional you wanted to say. Never say quick good nights. Linger, just as though you were expecting him to kiss you good night. Touch his leg or his arm fleetingly. You can pretend that you're falling asleep, and maybe get away with dropping your head on his shoulder. And almost any school boy can tell you that, if you somehow magically find yourself in a bed with him, the feigned sleep method is one sure way of making a pass without being obvious.

The bedroom, in any event, can be a fine place for playing upon his conditioned reflexes. You just know what his lower mind is going to be thinking of in connection with beds. You can wander into the bedroom while you're carrying on a very serious discussion, and even lounge on the bed. You can even accomplish almost the same result by lounging around on the floor. Lying down is more effective than sitting.

Tickling, and wrestling matches, are both ideal forms of body contact, that also utilize the conditioned reflex. With luck, you'll lose the match.

The massage is one of the best weapons in your arsenal. This gives you an opportunity to make contact with parts of his body you couldn't risk attacking directly, and if you handle it right, you can have him in a state of virtual undress.

Start with his shirt, and be businesslike about it all—no fair smirking. You want to relieve his aching muscles, and you can't do a good job for him with that cloth in the way. If he hesitates, you can even kid him about that—in other words, you're implying he's the one with dirty thoughts.

If he offers no resistance, suggest getting the trousers out of your way also, but if he balks, don't push the matter right off. Shrug, with a faint air of disgust at his lack of sobriety. You will, however, become more and more annoyed as the trousers keep getting in your way and making your task, which is only for his benefit anyway, more difficult. Work about the waist and try to get lower, saying as you clumsily attempt to knead the muscles under his belt, that this is one of the crucial areas of tension.

All the while, the massage really is working in your favor to relax him. The better you are at this, and it won't hurt to learn a little about massaging, the more relaxed you can make him, so that he will lazily obey when you finally ask, in a very discouraged voice, if he'll at least loosen his belt. Once he's done this, become bolder. Start back at the shoulders and quickly work your way to the waist again. This time keep going, under both the trousers and the shorts, as far as you can get. While you're at it, try pushing the trousers even further, as far as you can get them without protest.

The game is now in your hands, along with his backside. If you can coax him, without words, to let you pull the trousers down about his legs, he's practically your prisoner. In his relaxed state he'll probably not complain when you go to work upon his fanny and the backs of his legs; even if he did want to object, he's in rather an awkward position. Man is never less dignified than with his pants down about his ankles.

Get bolder, and at the same time less businesslike, as though the sight of his naked loveliness has started planting ideas in your mind, for the very first time. Let your hands tremble a little—they probably are anyway —breathe heavily, talk less. If he jumps up and starts rearranging his clothes, he needs more work. If he starts breathing heavily, you're ready to start massaging other things. This technique, by the way, will be easiest of all with the Athlete, who generally requires little coaxing to display his body.

Nearness is another important tool. Always make it a point to sit or stand close to him. Remember that thinking sexy is an aphrodisiac, so let your mind run rampant, and let a little of it show in your eyes. Talk in a low voice, so he'll have to stay close enough to hear you. Your eyes are on him, remember. Look up to him, literally. If he's not taller than you, try to arrange it so that he is seated higher than you. Your attitude is one of worshipful awe at being in his presence.

Every opportunity for intimacy is an opportunity to further your schemes. Brush the dust from his trousers, and be thorough about it. And ask him to brush your trousers—be sure to get lots of dust or fuzz on them, so he'll have to really work on them.

Get a cramp, and ask him to rub it for you to ease the pain, which is ghastly. If he's not much of a drinker, try getting him a little tipsy, or get high yourself, high enough that you need his help to un-dress and get into bed.

The more advanced example of this technique is the Necessary Intimacy approach, famous among straight Romeos for generations. For some amazing reason, these same Lotharios won't recognize this approach when it's used on them—until it's too late.

The spilled drink is the classic use of this technique, an extreme and bold approach, but quite often successful. Here you must really lay aside all your moral hesitations. The drink you want to spill is the sort that could cause a stain, for reasons which will be apparent. And I heartily recommend practicing this with a friend, substituting a glass of water.

Start by making the glass as difficult to hold as possible. Ideally, the glass will have straight up and down sides, harder to hold on to. You can wet the glass with water, or go even further and oil it slightly, not enough to be conspicuous, just enough to make it slick—try baby oil, a very thin film.

The idea, as you've guessed, is to accidentally spill

the drink on him. You should be slightly off balance, or looking elsewhere as you hand him the drink, so that you can let go of it before he has a good grip.

Of course, when it's spilled, you will be mortified and practically in tears. Humbly but firmly you'll insist that he remove his trousers while you take the stain out and dry them, which may take hours.

There is another highly successful variation of this technique, but one that you cannot necessarily plan far in advance, primarily because it depends upon circumstances such as the weather. But you can watch and be alert for the opportunities. Suppose, for instance, you're in the rainy season. Try to fix things so that you're caught out in the rain, without umbrellas and such. Whether you run for his apartment or yours makes little difference, assuming that both are equally private.

You'll have to take off those clothes to let them dry, and possibly take warm showers. If he's at your apartment, you won't think of letting him leave in the rain (hide your umbrella). If you are at his, be brave, ask if you can spend the night, explaining that you're already feeling chilled. Having planted that excuse, it won't seem strange when, soon after you're asleep beside him, you curl up against him for warmth.

The most drastic variation of this approach is the Stranded Together technique. For this one, you must shed your conscience completely. This is a last ditch stand, a do or die—in a manner of speaking.

You also need a bit of luck, or the right opportunity.

A snowstorm or rainstorm is ideal, if you can arrange it. Or you might arrange car trouble, if you're skilled enough to manage it and he's not skilled enough to spot it. Or you can interrupt a boating expedition by scuttling the boat while you're on that little island. Of course, it's up to you to figure out how to get yourselves rescued once your scheme has succeeded. The longer you keep him there with only you as a companion and outlet for his various urges, the more agreeable he will be—assuming, of course, you haven't fainted from malnutrition by then.

There are endless possibilities, and you must train yourself to be alert for them. Take advantage of practice, and be alert for that golden moment.

Two points worth mentioning before we finish this chapter. First, you should be prepared for anything once he succumbs to your wiles. I don't care how he acts out of bed, he may be just the opposite in bed. The terribly masculine sort who resisted homosexual advances for so long may not want to do a thing but lift his legs into the air, and that effeminate number you thought would spend his time with his face in the pillow may prove to be all man. If you expect to be successful, you've got to be prepared to keep him happy. You may be the very first who recognized and catered to his real nature, and he'll love you for it.

Another important part of "bedmanship," too often neglected, is the post-operative period. When it's done, don't try to talk about it, unless he brings the subject up. Don't worry, once the ice is broken, these things usually repeat themselves. Remember the things that won him—such as letting him be a man, and acting like one yourself—and keep them up. The sex is just an additional bonus you've offered him, not, so far as he should know, the goal you had in mind all the time. Forget about the others you've had, he's the first and only one. Don't get cutesy romantic, hold hands, or pinch him. Don't ask him if he hates you for what happened—once the suggestion is planted, he might decide to do just that—and don't walk around like a guilty murderer.

One last suggestion—talk is dangerous in a seduction. Never ask a man if you can kiss him, grope him, take him to bed, or anything of that sort. His modesty or uncertainty may prompt him to decline when, if you went ahead on the assumption that permission was yours, he'd offer no objection. If a man has to agree, he's making an accomplice of himself—he may not yet be ready for premeditated sex. Let him think it was an accident, or at least that he was overpowered. It's easier on his ego, at least the first few times. If he has to pretend to be very drunk or very sleepy, let him pretend—your rewards are still the same, and you know, or can certainly tell, that he's enjoying it just as much as you are. Keep your smirks to yourself and let him convince himself that he's calling the tune. We know better.

# CHAPTER TWELVE
## LABOR PAINS

NO, my dear—working, offices, employment, paychecks—that kind of labor pain. We all realize that they are necessary pains with which we're afflicted, but why not make them as pleasant as possible, and as productive?

At about eight o'clock on any morning, glance out your apartment window. See all those men moving around on the streets? They're going somewhere—somewhere away from the little woman and kiddies, the girl friend, and that sort of nonsense. They will be unattached for almost eight hours, maybe longer. You should be with them.

Even if you're an advocate of the "don't get your meat where you get your bread" philosophy, there's still no reason why you can't get them after the five o'clock whistle blows, or whatever blows at your place.

Let's think for a moment about your present employment. Are you happy on the job? If so, good for you—skip to the next chapter.

If not, what are you doing about it? Nothing, I'll bet. That paycheck has been paying the bills, and that's all that really matters, right? Wrong. Do you realize that almost a third of your life is spent on the job? If you're not enjoying yourself and bettering your life, you're wasting an awful lot of unhappy hours.

Make up your mind to do something about it. The easiest time to look for something new and interesting is when you have something dull and paying. There are plenty of job opportunities in the Sunday papers and there are an awful lot of employers who won't think twice about your using a few devious tactics to get a day off in order to appear for that interview.

Then, of course, while you're drudging along at that dull daytime job you could be looking into furthering your education and abilities with evening classes, as I suggested a few chapters back. The rewards are many. The best thing that ever happened to—well, let's call him Jack—was that he decided to go to one of the local universities' extension classes. Jack is about 45, so you can see he had quite a few reservations about applying for admission, knowing that most of the people there would be about half his age.

You'd be surprised at the results. Jack is now a confirmed believer in the powers of schooling. He not only has advanced in his job, but he made so many new acquaintances and adopted so many new outlooks and ideas, that he is no longer the old, dull Jack we all knew. He has more friends and broader views, and is a delightful change from the self-pitying, ready-for-the-grave type he once was.

What about your present job? Let's say you have a

position with no authority, maybe a billing clerk in a factory. The pay is okay, it pays for your modest apartment and the few luxuries you enjoy. The boss is fat, old and dreadfully anti-gay.

You're bored to tears, but afraid to change because you lack the self-confidence to better yourself. Well, grab your bootstraps and let's hike them up a bit. First of all, are there any other opportunities surrounding you to which you may advance? If so, ask for them. Don't just ask for a raise and be content with the same old routine. Chances are they'll think you are too dissatisfied if you merely ask for an increase in salary for the same old work output. Show them you want to improve your status. You're now ready to take on more responsibility, ask that they give you that chance. More money will come with the advance, as you become worth more.

Now if there aren't any openings to which you can climb, then do as I suggested previously—scan the newspapers and try to find something that offers a ladder to climb. For instance, get a typing job with the railroad; they are notorious for hiring male clerical help who ultimately fill the supervisory positions when they learn the work. The airlines offer good possibilities too. Typing jobs can often lead to far more interesting positions.

Don't forget those evening classes. Try to get yourself a trade—and I'm not referring to "that kind" of trade. Learn to be self-sufficient by developing the talents you have. A few years ago a young man I know decided to buy a poodle. During the first year and a half he had developed a breeding business that was more than just paying the bills. Today he has one of the best known kennels in Southern California and not only boards and breeds, but has learned to bathe and clip. He's doing extremely well because he liked dogs.

There are numerous ways of going into business for yourself, depending upon your individual interests, and your determination. Oh yeah, you say, but nowadays it's impossible to get started without help. As I say, that depends upon you. A few years back, David was slinging hash in a cheap restaurant. He wanted to work with flowers, as a designer, but he had checked around and found that no one was interested in hiring a person with no experience. Nor could he afford those expensive schools that give a lot of theory and little practice.

David decided to get his training from the experts, and pay for it with the two commodities he had to spare—time and energy. He went to the shops in the city and told them that he was willing to work for free, and work hard, on his Saturdays and free afternoons. In exchange, he asked only that he be allowed to watch the designer, and ask questions from time to time.

Needless to say, his offer was accepted, particularly when the shop had a lot of parties, or was in a busy season. For several months, David donated every evening and weekend to serving as an apprentice to many very excellent designers.

That's stupid, you say, I wouldn't work for nothing.

Well, maybe that's why you're still slinging hash, and David is now one of the finest and most successful designers in the field, with his own very respected shop.

Whatever your interests, you could do the same—cooking, fashion designing, commercial art—there are masters in all fields who would welcome a free lackey, and allow you to learn from them.

As for the financial backing necessary to start a business, if you show any initiative at all there are such places as the Small Business Administration, and most banks have small business loan departments that will help you. You may even find some individual to advance the money if your ideas are good enough and have promise. You'd be surprised at the number of people who are just waiting for some new ideas on which to put their money to work.

There's always hustling, if you have the face and body for it. I'll warn you, there's no future in it, and the work gets pretty dull after a while. But any hobby may be the key to your successful future. Give some thought to making it pay, even if the pay is small to begin; sometimes it does take years to get it really going. I have another friend who earns his living in the display field. His real interest, though, is painting and sculpting. Over the years, he's been keeping his hobby up, evenings and weekends, selling pieces when he could. Now, after many years, he's ready to devote full time to his art work.

Of course, not everyone has the sort of talent necessary, or is temperamentally suited to having his own business. But you can still have the kind of job that expresses you, and allows you to prosper, mentally and financially. For one thing, consider the type of establishment in which you're going to spend all those hours. Another thing, are you suited to it? For another, are the men the sort who interest you?

If you like the young, aggressive, masculine, semi-straight men, for instance, why not apply at the engineering firms or architectural offices. On the other hand I know many good, hard-working, well-paid gays who work for trucking firms and shipping companies, and manage incidentally to make out quite well with the local talent, although they don't let it interfere with their work output. Let's be honest, wouldn't it be more fun to have your coffee breaks surrounded by the dream-type men you admire so? Even if you can't touch right then and there, think of all the groundwork you'll be laying. You just may end up laying some of your co-workers.

You can't be serious, working in an office full of elderly women. It may increase your popularity with older women, but I hope they aren't your goal.

Banks make excellent places for starting in the business world. I know more gay bankers than anyone, and believe me, tellers can climb pretty far up if they put their minds to it. Besides, think about the contacts you'll be making. Use your winning smile and personality on the ten-to-three customers, and not only they but your supervisor will notice you and mark you for that raise or advancement you are actually striving for.

Don't scoff at being a ribbon clerk, either. I know some pretty important buyers and managers who started out by selling shirts and ties. Then again, don't work for a women's shop. Chances are most of your contacts will be women. Try for the local haberdasher—it's much more interesting helping the fitter in a men's shop than in a lady's. And think of the customers—even the most heavenly creature has to buy his trousers somewhere.

If you have itchy feet, why not try the travel business. The money isn't too good to start off, but think of all the horizons it opens up for you. I can't think of one boring or dull travel agent—well, not very many anyway. The fringe benefits are gigantic after the first year or two.

You may like to read. Fine, why not develop that into a career? There are publishing companies and editors who employ part-time readers—and while you're earning that part-time money you can be going to school during your other hours, training for that profession you want so badly.

You have a good speaking voice—offer your services to the Foundation for the Blind, reading aloud or making records for the blind. You'd be surprised where it can lead you.

Maybe you're a camera bug. Try for those contests you see advertised in the monthlies. The same goes for writing skills. I started as a hobby writer, many years ago in junior high school. I wrote mystery stories, featuring myself and my classmates, and it helped make me popular—everyone wanted to get into the act. Strangely enough, when school was over, I wasted many years on dull office jobs, before I even thought of developing my writing into a career. I can't afford to drive a Rolls Royce, and I have yet to win my first Nobel Prize, but I earn a comfortable income doing something I enjoy.

There's another matter to be considered, the you that is presented to the outside world. I've already touched on mannerisms, affectations, and make-up. If you're the frivolous, obvious type who has trouble getting work in an office, or trouble getting a job anywhere, I have only one suggestion—tone yourself down. Even if you happen to land that job as receptionist in the local beauty parlor, no one, and I stress no one, will be too interested in you or your problems if your arms are constantly waving and your eyes are made up to look like Cleopatra's.

What if you enjoy your present job, but you can't see much future in it? Ask yourself why there isn't any future. Is it your fault or the fault of management? If it's truly the latter, then I still suggest you consider a change. But be honest in stating that the fault isn't yours.

Perhaps you haven't been taking that long, serious look at yourself before starting out for the office in the morning. Don't laugh at those bad breath commercials. Don't wear that silly sports jacket and beat-up looking pair of trousers again today. It's better to wear one nice-looking suit every day, as a young friend of mine did for a year, than to change off each day and continue looking bad, if different.

Improve your appearance. If your voice is a hindrance, do what I suggested before and work on lowering it. Buy a tape recorder, and read aloud into it. Listen, and decide how to improve it. Find a pleasant speaking register and practice reading and talking aloud, until that voice becomes natural to you.

If there are opportunities on the job for you, see to it that you get them. Don't let that new fellow who was hired last week get that new opening you had your eye on.

What about personality clashes? Is it all the other person's fault, or are you being a little difficult? Are you practicing your warm regard?

Don't sit around feeling sorry for yourself because the guy in the next apartment got a raise and is heading for New York as manager of his firm's new office. He worked to get that new position; find out how he did it and follow in his footsteps. Most people are flattered to be asked for the secret of their success. If he happens to be a Desirable and an Available, so much the better—you're working on his ego, and maybe establishing a nice relationship in addition to improving yourself.

Another cardinal rule—don't carry your work problems home with you. Work should be done at work, even if it means staying at the office an extra thirty minutes—not at the local pub, crying on a friend's shoulder. You'll wind up crying alone.

Now, are you thoroughly convinced of what you're

going to do? I hope so. I've tried my best to tug at those bootstraps for you. The rest is up to you. Pull hard, and let's get going. The only way, in this regard, is going up. Going down is reserved for something else.

# CHAPTER THIRTEEN
## A CLEAN GETAWAY

NO ONE likes to be turned down or left at the altar. Then, on the other hand, you may say, "So what?" If you happen to be the one turning them down or leaving them flat. But think a minute. Haven't there been those instances when you've said that fatal "no" to someone at first meeting and regretted it afterward? Or haven't you ever been guilty of breaking off a love affair with someone whom you really would have liked to retain as a friend? We all have, so don't feel too badly. But what I'd like to try to do is give you a few pointers as to how to turn them down so that no feelings are hurt and you come out smelling like Gertrude Stein's rose is a rose is a...

A few years ago I had a love affair afloat and suddenly for no reason at all I started to become disinterested. I knew it was proving to be an unworkable situation, and we finally split. Then one day soon afterward I ran into my ex-beau in company with an extremely handsome young man and it got me to thinking. Did I really break it off or was he so tactful and used such excellent strategy that he made me think I was the one who walked out? I fretted about it for quite a while before I realized that I had been associated with one of the smartest men around.

There lies the secret to the successfully breaking off of an affair. Get him to say good-bye to you, by using a little forethought and planning your escape carefully. You'll wind up with his respect and that of your friends, rather than having CAD painted all over you.

It does take some scheming, and some of the tactics are unquestionably devious. If you prefer to take the more direct approach, fine. Sometimes the very best method is simply to face him bluntly and say you want to call quits. If he's the reasonable type who will take this in stride and accept your offer of continued friendship, then this is certainly the method I recommend.

Not all lovers are this reasonable. You may instead wind up with a tantrum on your hands, or a scene, and finally give in and agree to try again, even though your heart isn't in it. If your lover and your relationship are the sort that make this seem likely, then I suggest using a more devious approach. In that case, there are certain methods almost guaranteed to do the trick.

Lesson 1. Be late—I mean like an hour or so. When you do show, don't explain. He'll burn and sizzle, and finally demand an explanation. At this point, you will be angered by his distrust. As you storm out, throw him a parting explanation: "I had to take my mother to the hospital," or, "I stopped to get tickets to the opera you wanted to see." He'll feel like two cents, but too late, you've already slammed the door.

Lesson 2. Be a slob—but only for his benefit and never when other people can see you. For example, you've gone to his home for dinner. He's taken every pain to prepare a lovely meal, and you fall asleep before finishing the first cocktail. Then, when you're awakened for dinner by a surly host, you're not really hungry. After picking over the food, you leave early. You can make it worse by dropping food, spilling gravy, upsetting wine glasses, and such.

Lesson 3. More sleep—yawn a lot and go the early-to-bed-early-to-rise routine. You have to get up early. You worked late at the office. You feel a cold coming on. You're on a health kick that requires you to get ten hours of sleep every night—anything that gives you an excuse to go to bed early. For heaven's sake, don't go tricking as soon as you drop him off. He may walk into the same bar, and you've come out a heel, instead of with a clean bill of health.

Lesson 4. You are broke—no money for anything, not even that $.15 beer he suggests you stop for. Your job is insecure, the rent is overdue, the boss just cut your salary, you have too many doctor bills. Cry the money blues until he turns blue with cold. When he calls the relationship off, he'll look awfully silly telling your friends he left you because you had no money.

Lesson 5. You are sick, all the time—colds, flu, viruses, high blood pressure, bad liver, prostate infections, kidney stones—anything that will restrict your social activities. No cocktails before dinner, no staying up late, no sex. Get the idea? Unless he turns out to be Florence Nightingale, you're out. No one enjoys playing doctor and nurse all the time.

Lesson 6. If he's the indoor type, reverse the above procedure. You're late because you had to play that set of tennis after work. Exercise is your first love. Walking, running, swimming, anything that keeps you out of doors.

Lesson 7. If he's not the bookish or intellectual sort, philosophize about everything. Spout off constantly about Schopenhauer, hum or whistle off pitch and tell him it is Schoenberg or Shostakovich. Be a snob, always comparing him with obscure literary characters. Find fault with everything he says, or just plainly disagree with him and point out your own reverse philosophies on the subject.

Lesson 8. Again, reverse the procedure if he is an intellectual. Acquire an interest in rock and roll, beatnik poetry, or anything you know he'll dislike. Buy him some Elvis Presley records and insist he play them when you're around. And make it look as though you really dig the stuff. If he mentions the concert you attended recently, tell him you no longer dig that fruit music.

Always, always make certain that you handle it with finesse and tact. Even being insulting can be done properly, but make sure the insult has hit its target before you try soothing it over. And remember, not too soothing. Just a light touch is the right touch.

A few years ago a friend was living with a lover, a very handsome creature who idolized my friend. My friend, however, had begun to tire of seclusion, and wanted to get back into the swing of things, while his lover cared only for sailboats, and lonely beaches. It was over, and should have been ended promptly.

My friend made a mistake. He began to drink, partially to annoy his teetotaler lover. In an attempt to soothe troubled waters, his lover began joining him. Not only were the two of them drinking themselves silly, but after the first drink each evening, they would begin quarreling. In a short time, they had learned to hate one another.

They did decide finally to split up, a mutual decision, but by this time my friend found there was nothing he could do to retain a friendship. He knew, of course, that sex was a dead issue, but he really did enjoy his ex-lover's company out of bed, and thought he was a fine person. To his chagrin, however, his ex wouldn't even answer his phone. He wanted nothing, absolutely nothing, to do with my friend.

Unfortunate, but not an unusual occurrence. Next time you find yourself with a failing romance, give some thought to the suggestions above before snatching up that train ticket to Reno.

Another important point. Whatever you do when trying to break off an affair, don't ever drag friends, relations, or innocent bystanders into the problem. You'll regret it ever afterward—if, that is, you still have any friends, relations, or innocent bystanders when the smoke finally settles. You'd be surprised how easily you can lose friends by involving them in your quarrels. It's bad business; don't bankrupt yourself by making that mistake.

So much for breaking off the marriage or engagement. But there are other occasions when you're out for an evening, and someone decides the two of you were meant for one another, but you don't share the opinion. He's not your type, or he has two heads, or you're not in the mood, or whatever, but you want to avoid his advances. How do we handle that?

The first and probably most effective solution is to play it cool—and I mean frosted, with icicles hanging from your earlobes. This doesn't mean you have to be insulting. For all you know, he might turn out to be your boss's brother, or your best friend's new roommate—or he may prove to be with a very lovely friend. Be polite, but distant, and whatever you do, don't encourage it

A good friend of mine is the type person who can't discourage anyone and hates to hurt people's feelings. I saw him standing in a bar one night with a real yo-yo, who was pawing and making over my friend. Friend just stood there and soaked it in like a Greek sponge in a downpour. Whether or not he was enjoying the pawing and fawning I don't know, but what I do know is that a perfectly fantastic specimen of manhood sitting next to me on the stool remarked about good-looking friend and Mr. Yo-yo. The fellow next to me had been interested in friend, but he became very disinterested on seeing friend's apparent taste. My friend struck out, without even knowing he was in the game.

A good trick I learned to use when they get too pushy—and we all have had occasion to try to fend off some pushy number who won't take no for an answer— is to merely hold a drink or a cigarette between me and him. He won't take the chance of getting his chin burned or a drink spilled on him. And it keeps him at that safe distance, which will allow your head and eyes to turn, scanning the room for an escape route or a rescue party.

In that vein, if you have a good friend (by now you should), consider a pact. When you're out cruising and one of you meets up with an undesirable, the other will immediately rescue you by coming up and playing the role of jealous lover. I have used this successfully many times. Do, by the way, have an agreed-upon signal— his idea of undesirable may not coincide with yours, and he may be chasing away someone you were really interested in talking to. Chances are, when you use this technique, that Mr. Undesirable will apologize to both of you, thereby winning your respect with no feelings trampled into the dust.

Of course, there are other methods you can use. If you're the type who can get away with it, drop an accidental hint that you are a member of the local vice team. That'll scare even the bravest of them.

Another method, and the simplest, is to excuse yourself politely and walk to the other side of the bar or room. If he follows you, simply tell him you're cruising someone else. In most cases, he'll respect your wishes.

Naturally you can pull the "I'm married and true"

bit, but chances are he'll only persist, knowing that you're out without the other half. Of course, you can tell him you're waiting for hubby to show, but when you leave soon afterward with that number who's been sitting two stools down the bar, you've made a liar out of yourself, and an enemy out of him.

The very best discouragement is silence—utter, complete, and definite silence. Nothing—no smile, no comment, no look—no reaction at all. Just pretend no one spoke. He'll get the message.

While I'm on the subject of utter silence, I'd like to throw in another tip. Silence pertains particularly in the unhappy situation of meeting up with Mr. Vice Squad. A very good friend of mine was accosted lately in the men's room of a gasoline station. He was having his car filled with gas and decided to relieve himself before starting his long trek home. When he went in he found three urinals, two of which were occupied, leaving the center one free. Being somewhat shy he tried in vain to do what was necessary, which caused him to linger at the urinal waiting for the two gentlemen to finish.

When they didn't, my friend decided to forget it and go on his way. He knew that one gentleman was cruising him, but he also knew that the entire neighborhood was frequently patrolled by vice squad.

My friend wasn't interested in the one cruising him, who was too effeminate for his tastes, but he was always one to do a good deed. When they chanced to reach the exit at almost the same time, my friend said in a low voice, "Don't you know this area is hot?"

That was all he needed to say—a few weeks and $600.00 later, that comment had been officially recorded as, "I only live a few blocks from here." In fact, my friend lived quite a distance away, but vice officers are not committed to facts. In making the remark that he did, my friend had confirmed the officer's suspicion that he was homosexual, and marked himself as fair game for an arrest. The men count on the fact that most homosexuals cannot or will not defend themselves. The best rule to follow in such a situation is silence, total and complete. Even a simple "excuse me" is too much to risk. By the time you get to court, that may have become, "It's you, the man I love."

There are other situations in which it is necessary to do some ducking. You may even find it necessary to dodge someone in whom you are interested, because for one reason or another he's genuinely unavailable. For instance, your best friend comes over with his newest love for an evening of bridge. The new lover takes to you like moths to a flame and the footsie game begins under the table. This new number is lovely, and you'd give a month's salary for just one night of love.

The first thing to consider is which is more important, your sex life or the friendship. Even if it's the former, you still have problems. Once word gets around that you snatch tricks from under noses, your doorbell will be ringing less and less, and you'll lose one of the most valuable sources of new material, your friends.

If that isn't important to you either, then go ahead and be the cad you are—your ex-friend will understand, and never speak to you again.

The situation can be handled nicely, however, in a number of ways. First, you have to start by ending the footsies. If possible though, before tucking your feet safely under your chair, kick off a shoe and run your foot lightly over the trick's foot. This way, he knows that you too are interested, in the event of a future meeting. At the same time, with only one light touch, you're not making yourself too available. We all know that some people just test everyone they meet to see if they are available, and lose interest as soon as that's established. By leaving him hanging slightly, you'll keep him interested.

If your friend is a really good one, things are easy for you. Get him alone in the kitchen and ask how serious his feelings are. He may tell you to be his guest. If he doesn't, you can still ask him to let you know when he's finished with it.

If that doesn't seem like a safe approach, depending upon the friend, you'll have to wait until they are ready to leave. At this time, it will be perfectly proper to shake the new trick's hand. Squeeze it firmly and warmly, look him straight in the eyes with just the right message in yours, and say you hope you'll see him again real soon. He should get the message, and if he's really interested, he'll get in touch. In that line, a friend of mine makes it quite simple to stay in touch. He keeps a "guest register" by the door, and it's a rule of the house that everyone signs it, so your friend can't accuse you. Also, he keeps a small dish of calling cards near the door, with his own name and phone number on them, which he customarily hands to departing guests. In this way, he has their number, and they have his.

There are other situations that present themselves. Let's say you're at a party and a bore is occupying all your time and preventing you from circulating. You can't be rude because the bore is the host's lover and recently broke his leg in a skiing accident and is confined to the couch. He thinks you're fun to talk with and doesn't realize he's monopolizing your entire evening and cutting your chances to nothing.

First thing you do is excuse yourself to go to the bathroom or to get yourself another drink, or offer to fetch him something. Then you try your best to approach your host with the problem, honestly and directly. If you feel that your direct approach to the host will only cause more hurt feelings, then don't risk it. Instead, linger with a group you find interesting. Linger long enough to coax someone you like to join you on the couch with invalid co-host. Or search out someone else to take your place on the couch, doing it tactfully.

I found myself in a similar situation when an East Coast friend called to say that one of his best friends was coming to the West Coast, and would I do everything possible to entertain him. I called in friends and prepared what should have been a lovely evening. Alas, this visitor was not only dull, but obnoxious and insulting. My first reaction was to take a saber to him, but I remembered my promise to my friend. So I gathered my closest friends into the kitchen for a war conference. Out of consideration for me (you see, you do need all those friends I've been encouraging you to collect), it was agreed that we would all take shifts talking with the visitor. Each person spent as long with him as he could bear, then signaled another to take his place. It worked, and left the rest of us free to have a nice evening.

Finally, I'll give you an example of how one expert managed to duck a particular problem. He happens to be quite a good pianist. Whenever we were invited to parties, poor he was usually asked to play and, being a good guest, he consented. Regrettably, he ended up spending all his time at the piano and missing all the fun.

After numerous parties and numerous complaints, we hit upon a scheme. My voice is pretty dreadful, and I don't mind admitting the fact. So the very next party, he seated himself and rattled off something short and sweet. When encores were called for, as usual, he insisted he would play only if I would sing. It took only one song. At the next party, we repeated the performance. Soon, requests for his playing had dropped to a bare minimum.

Ducking, dodging, and ditching are arts. They can be done, and to your advantage. A clean getaway is an essential part of the gay world. Don't leave those nasty scars. Tire tracks after a hit-and-run have caught many an offender.

# CHAPTER FOURTEEN
## SILVER THREADS
## AMONG THE GOLD

NO, don't skip over this chapter, even if you are only twenty-one and just had your first legal beer at the local pub. Middle age will get to you eventually, be assured. You might as well start preparing for it.

What do you consider middle age? Well, ask any twenty-year-old and he'll tell you thirty. Ask a thirty-year-old and he'll tell you forty. Never ask a forty-year-old.

Whatever age marks the border, when you get to that "natures spelled backwards" point, you've arrived, and Serutan isn't the whole solution. If it makes you feel better, of course, go right ahead and stock up on it—and while you're at it, take stock of yourself.

No, the ball isn't over for you. There's still quite a bit of living to do, so don't drag out the pet hound and slippers and retire to the fireside, unless you've found that lifelong companion already.

If you've already gone the slippers route, get out of them right now and put them in mothballs—you've got work to do. Old fairies don't fly away, they turn into charming, above-reproach godmothers, bringing joy and happiness to all the poor little Cinderellas sitting around by the hearths—and in the doing, manage to get their own ashes taken care of. Got your wand ready?—no, the one with the star on the top. Off we go, into the wild, wild, wild, blown yonder.

You're at that unmentionable age, and you're feeling it, right? That's your first mistake. Don't let it get you down or you'll have everyone convinced that you are old. First rule—never remind people of how old you are. Believe it or not they'll start believing you, and nothing will unconvince them once you've proved it by your constant complaining. There will be those days when you'll search for pity, and bemoan your lost youth. Do us both a favor—stay home alone on those days, away from everyone. Don't succumb to that malicious urge to point out your sagging skin and wrinkles. Your friends will notice them forever after, even at the party when you're feeling 25 again. It's a subject strictly for you, and one not to be shared, not even with your older friends. Always remember, they are older than you—even if they are not. Think young, and you'll be surprised at how much better you'll feel and do.

Good advice—don't think for one moment that dressing like a youngster will make you look young. It will only serve to make you look ridiculous, and emphasize your age. No one thinks an old auntie in tight pants and plaid cap looks sexy. Silly, yes, but definitely undesirable. And that goes for the little red hotrod with the top back and some fat, silly old queen at the wheel in her jockey helmet, and for the motorcycle bit. If you happen to be the type that digs the aging leatherette, go to it, but I personally look upon them as foolish. Not even that movie star we all know can manage to look sexy in those things at his age. Now a middle-aged man in a trucker's outfit is something else, but only when he's driving that truck. He looks the part that he's playing, not like he's out for Halloween.

All right, speaking of truckers, consider this. You're happily married to that gorgeous hulk of middle age and he comes home from his long jaunt on the highway. Sexy, right? Now, after he's had his shower and cleaned up and you want to go out for a nice dinner, wouldn't you really prefer to be escorted by that same lovely male, attired in a trim-fitting pair of slacks, dark blazer, and open-neck shirt? You see, you've gotten both in one marvelous, middle age package. Incredible, you say? Not at all, I'm describing the lover of a very good friend—one of the sexiest men I know. He has taken advantage of all the experience and training that he's had time to acquire, so that he can now adapt himself to almost any environment. That's taking advantage of his middle age, turning a handicap into an asset.

Before you get too despondent over your age, study those handsome, virile male leads on the silver screen. With few exceptions, those attractive men who set hearts aflutter are well into the middle-age bracket. You don't see them starving for attention, or dying of loneliness. And they're not all that beautiful either—sexy, yes.

Now, back to those of you who are already middle-age packages. No one, you'll say, wants an old queen. My answer to that is, don't be an old queen. Be a man—not the rough and tough Forest Ranger sort, unless that's your nature, but a real, honest to goodness, charming, delightfully suave, polished man. You can do it. You have all the experience now. You've been at the game for years, so you know the pitfalls to look for. You know the art of sex and love, and how to entertain and be charming. You have an edge on the market, whether you realize it or not.

There will be times when you're really hot after that smart little twenty-three-year-old blond sitting next to you at the party and lo and behold, he's gone off with another twenty-three-year-old before the party has ended. No, wait a minute, reflect. Would he have gone home with you if you had been twenty-three? Possibly, and possibly not. You might not have been his type to begin with, in which case your age was not the real reason. And why did he sit and talk with you in the first place? He must have found something attractive or interesting, or he wouldn't have wasted his time. Lovely young twenty-three-year-olds are not famous for wasting their time. Was it your charm, your maturity, your common sense and sensibility?

Maybe you started telling him what was wrong with the youth of today, and that it takes age and maturity to really learn what life is all about. Did you let your superiority complex show? That's where you lost out, then. Youth doesn't want to learn all about life second hand, at one sitting. They want to live it and experience it. No one could tell you, when you were at that age, what you were doing wrong and how you would regret it someday. You got bored with it as soon as they started.

Don't go to the other extreme, either, by trying to make yourself over into a twenty-three-year-old because you're with one. I've already warned you about that. They're with you because they happen to want a little maturity to lean on in case of fire, and fires are frequent in their lives.

Think about the ancient Greeks. Their society was founded on the young boy-older man relationship. And that tendency has carried through right down to the present age, in many subtle forms. Today we have the Boy Scouts, and Big Brother—every boy, they say, needs a man.

Now let's be brutal about things. With middle age comes the necessity of doubling your efforts, and working harder. You've reached the time of life when time is a factor—the time you spend on all night dancing and drinking bouts. Get to bed earlier from time to time, to keep those shadows and lines to a minimum. Diet is important, as well as exercise. Both are dirty words, I know, but absolutely necessary evils as far as you're concerned. There is nothing that will make you look older than a spreading waistline or flabbiness. Keep those muscles toned up—go to a gym. It may be more fun than you think.

Watch what you eat and stay away from those hot fudge sundaes and malted milks. I know they're delicious, but so are those lovely young things you're working for.

You're probably able to hold more liquor now than the youthful members of the bar, but don't try to show off. Even if you do succeed in remaining sober, those extra pounds will show up sooner or later. Try to keep drinking to a minimum.

Gravity has been pulling at you for a good many years and there's no way of reversing the poles, but there are a few helpful hints.

Start with the hair—how do you like it? Is it thin on top? Well, there are several solutions. There's the hairpiece we talked about before. Or, a good barber or hair stylist can advise you about coloring in the scalp to cover the thinness. These can be expensive, but by now you should have been on the job long enough to be successful at it. If not, you've at least acquired a little sensibility in managing your finances.

Money brings us to a painful subject—paying for your numbers. Personally, the out and out purchase is never a very appealing date. On the other hand, spare me your tirades. Even the young suitor pays for it in one way or another—by dinners, gifts, and work. Why should you be different? You should expect to pick up his dinner check, or buy him a drink. If he's the decent sort, he'll probably insist on buying you a drink in return. Of course, he can't afford to be lavish, but it's the token that's important. And as far as I'm concerned, spending money in this respect is not different than any other. The big question is still, are you getting your money's worth.

When others complain about an older man keeping a handsome youth, I disagree in silence. Chances are the man is getting far more enjoyment out of this expenditure than he would from a new car or a long vacation. So long as both parties are getting what they want and need out of the arrangement, who's to complain? No, I'm not trying to persuade you to find a paid companion. What I am saying is that you shouldn't regret paying for a dinner, in exchange for the company of an attractive, charming young man, and possibly a night of pleasure.

In the same vein, gifts are important. I don't mean that if he's a struggling pianist, you must send him a new Steinway. That's ridiculous, and will only mark you in his opinion as a crass lecher. But if he happens to mention a poem he likes, or interest in a particular subject, don't be afraid to pick up a book on it and present it to him the next time you see him. You'll be amazed at the dividends it pays, better than most blue chips.

Don't ever forget that those young lovelies surround themselves with a group of their same age bracket, just as you do. Those young friends of his can't afford to do some of the things you do, such as buying tickets to that show they all want to see so badly. Aren't you being impressive when you call and his roommate answers the phone, and you leave a message to let him know, as well as his friends, that you would like to take him to that special show? Have tickets on hand for those really good things coming up, which you bought in advance, before it was sold out. You'll not only impress your trick, and give him something to crow about, but you've also made his roommates susceptible to your advances, if you change your mind about him.

Back to appearance. If you happen to be silver-haired and hate it, do something about it. Personally I love silver temples on a man. I think they make him look distinguished. Who cares for distinguished men, you ask? All those lovely young things, if you must know, or at least a big percentage of them. Call it father-complex, brother-complex, or what you like— the important thing is that they are attracted to you.

Regardless of their underlying psychological motives, they still want to go to bed with you. And isn't it fortunate, your sex technique is much more advanced than theirs. Show them how it should be done—they'll be back for seconds, thirds, or sixty-ninths.

If those bags under your eyes are another bothersome detail, there are remedies. Mind you, a recent survey revealed that women found men with bags under their eyes sexier. Unfortunately, I can't say how well that applies to young men and their reactions. In any case, you can spend a few hundred dollars to have them removed. There's even a cheaper solution. Before you go out, crack an egg and separate the white into a cup. Dip your finger into the white and coat the sagging bag with it. Let it dry, about ten minutes, and voila, the bags have tightened up and almost disappeared. They'll stay that way for over an hour, at which time you'll feel the dryness. Just stick a finger in your mouth and moisten the hardened egg-white. Again it will contract and you can repeat it all night until the white has totally worn off.

By then you should have snagged that trick anyway and be safely snug in your bed, with the lights out. And by the way, I hope you're careful about the lights in your apartment. They should be soft and indirect. Harsh overhead lights will age you faster than a Dorian Grey with a slashed portrait. Candlelight is your best bet, whenever possible. Otherwise, you'll use a soft, pink bulb.

There are ointments on the market that do much the same thing as the egg whites, but the eggs work as well, and are much cheaper. You can return your cup to the refrigerator, with a little cellophane wrap over it, and continue using it for days.

There are commercial products such as Erase, which are intended to hide the shadows. However, they are chalky and noticeable, and look just like what they are—make-up.

As for suntans, they will only tend to dry and wrinkle the skin all the more. Unless you're going for that leathery, coarse effect, keep your sun-sessions to a minimum.

Now if you have all kinds of money and really want to de-wrinkle, there are two definite routes you can take. One is to have the face lifted. Before you consider this, however, you should be warned that face lifting is a major, serious operation, and you are endangered by possible damage to nerves, uneven lifting, hemorrhaging, and other problems. The cost will be in the neighborhood of $1,000.00, for which they cannot guarantee results. Further, you can have your face lifted more than once, but probably no more than three times.

The second possibility is called dermabrasion. It's also expensive, about $500.00 to $1,000.00, but much safer than surgery. Your local dermatologist will start by freezing the skin with a chemical spray, then he'll sand away the outer layer of skin with a softly rotating brush. Don't expect to display the results at once; you'll have to go into absolute hiding for a while. The face will scab over for several days, and then turn a nice lobster red. In a week or so, it will clear up, and the wrinkles will have practically disappeared. According to the medical reports I have read, patients are highly pleased with the results.

There is a third alternative—rejuvenation by injection. You can visit clinics in Switzerland, Germany, or England for treatments of this sort, many of them involving procaine. A famous actor, so I'm told, makes his pilgrimage regularly, and if he's an example of what can be done, he's a persuasive example. He's managed to look age thirty for more years than I care to calculate. You must be warned, however, this is quite expensive. A couple of thousand will probably see you through. And it's not recognized by the American medical society. In other words, although many people swear by it, you're still making a guinea pig of yourself.

Then of course you can have your blood cleaned, or even resort to black magic. Personally, I think your best remedy is to accept your fate and learn to use it to your best advantage. A desirable man remains a desirable man, at any age. Be sensible and utilize your wit and knowledge. Put the candles on the cake, but don't eat more than a sliver of the cake.

You'll be happier when you think healthy and positively. It's been said, and accurately, that age and growing old is not a matter of years, but of outlook. Try new hobbies and foods, continue looking for everything that's fresh, new, and exciting in life. Don't sink into those pits of gloom and despair—they can prove to be lonely and uncomfortable graves. I can't think of a single person who would voluntarily join you.

When afflicted with a bad mood, stay home alone—don't expose it to others. Cry for yourself, wallow in self-pity—and tomorrow, get busy and start improving your lot. There's no harm in being another day older—if you're also a day wiser.

# CHAPTER FIFTEEN
## WITCHES AND BITCHES, HEXES AND SEXES

A LOT of hog wash, you say. Well, there are an awful lot of people who believe in fairies, and an awful lot of fairies who believe in people. Who's to say what's right?

If someone walked up to you, a perfect stranger, and said "Aren't you a Gemini?" wouldn't you be flattered and interested, even if you knew nothing about astrology. I pooh-poohed that sort of thing for years, until exactly that thing happened to me. I don't recall how accurate the person was, but the important thing was, he had found an ingenious way to strike up a conversation with me, and capture my interest.

Many persons won't even speak to someone who was born under the wrong astrological sign. This is silly, to my thinking. Just for amusement, I consulted the charts on several of my friends and acquaintances, and found that they weren't supposed to like me at all. One I've lived with for the past many years, and the other is my oldest and best friend. We certainly don't let a little thing like a couple of stars, too far away to see clearly, spoil our relationships.

Be that as it may, I thought you might be interested in knowing a little about the various signs. The next number you start to work on may be a believer. Here, then, are a few things that the experts have to say, translated into our field of interest:

## March 21 to April 20—ARIES

You are bold, impulsive, and active. You have a tendency to exaggerate, and even just plain fib. Tact is not one of your strong points, yet you succeed in just about everything you attempt, so you have no excuse for not utilizing the suggestions I've given you in this book. Arians feel that everything natural is right. Stay away from Cancer, Libra and Capricorn. Your best bets are Taurus, Gemini, Leo, Sagittarius, Aquarius, and Pisces.

## April 21 to May 20—TAURUS

You are patient and willing to work, but you possess a terrible stubborn streak—bull-headedness, it's called. You are somewhat conservative in most things, slow, careful, steady, practical, and reserved. With those traits, seduction should be an easy hobby for you. Your most negative quality is that stubbornness, often blind to reasoning. Gemini, Cancer, Pisces, Virgo, Capricorn, and Aries are most compatible. But you will not get along with Leo, Scorpio, or Aquarius.

## May 21 to June 20—GEMINI

Intelligent, ambitious, sensitive and active. Talented, beautiful, powerful, sexy, wonderful, magnetic, personable, charming, witty, clever, logical, romantic—oh, I could just go on and on. I'm a Gemini. Some so-called authority claims that Gemini's are fragile and need a strong arm to lean on. Sheer nonsense, ask any of the many friends who lend me their support. We aren't supposed to like Virgo (my best friend is one), Sagittarius or Pisces. We get along very well with Cancer (he is a Cancer), Leo, Libra, Aquarius, Aries, and Taurus.

## June 21 to July 20—CANCER

He, in my case, is a Cancer, so I'm prejudiced here also. They are romantic, flirty, handsome, sensitive and artful—in or out of bed. They also usually end up spoiled rotten, but no one ever seriously objects. They get along best with Gemini, Leo, Virgo, Scorpio, Pisces, Taurus, and should never associate with Libra, Capricorn or Aries (I told him that last flirtation wouldn't work out).

## July 21 to August 21—LEO

Aristocratic, dependable, loyal, you Leos make excellent friends. You are honest, trustworthy, and have a good capacity for loving—often. Your greatest weakness is arrogance and your deep concern for your own marvelous opinion of yourself. That, and your pride, can sometimes make you unpopular, but even though you're snobs, you're usually nice snobs. You get along best with Virgo, Libra, Sagittarius, Aries, Gemini, and Cancer. Stay away from Scorpio, Aquarius, and Taurus.

### August 22 to September 22—VIRGO

Practical, thorough, methodical, and exact, you love small, minute detail. You like to criticize, which you do in the spirit of helpfulness, and are usually a very down-to-earth type person. Your most negative quality is that you are too cautious, to the point of timidity, and sometimes that wit of yours isn't funny at all, but cold and ironical. You should mingle with Libra, Scorpio, Capricorn, Taurus, Cancer, and Leo. But stay clear of Sagittarius, Gemini, and Pisces.

### September 23 to October 22—LIBRA

If the one you're after is Libra, you have a good chance —he has a predilection for homosexuality. He also has a love of harmony, and justice, and sympathy for pain and suffering (try getting sick). He's also sociable, charming, and companionable. He seldom leads a solitary life, and is serene, temperate, intellectual, and analytical, as well as even tempered. He may also be spineless and find it hard to take a firm attitude in hostile circumstances. He'd rather avoid any kind of unpleasantness at all costs, so avoid that scene. He'll get along with you best if you are Scorpio, Sagittarius, Aquarius, Gemini, Leo, and Virgo. He won't get along well with Capricorn, Aries, or Cancer.

October 23 to November 22—SCORPIO

You are an extremist in every way. You love mad, wild, uninhibited, almost debased things, you wild thing you. You are decisive in word and deed, indispensable to humanity, earnest and brave. Yet, you have a sort of vicious strength and daring intensity, and are capable of cunning and even cruelty. Made happy by all this should be Sagittarius, Capricorn, Pisces, Cancer, Virgo, and Libra. Scorpios don't mix well with Aquarius, Taurus, or Leo.

November 23 to December 20—SAGITTARIUS

High standards, mature outlook, far-seeing, and imaginatively practical. You are broad-minded, tolerant, humorous, and truthful, sympathetic, and affectionate. Your weakness lies in being lazy and boastful, but people will still consider you a pretty decent individual. Inconsiderate behavior is your worst fault, and you are sometimes tactless. You should surround yourself with Capricorn, Aquarius, Aries, Leo, Libra, Scorpio. Keep away from Pisces, Gemini, and Virgo.

## December 21 to January 19—CAPRICORN

You are ambitious, strong willed and definite in purpose. Loyalty and devotion are your strong points.

You have unbounded charm and are dignified and reserved. You have a fine mind, slow but capable of deep concentration. You hate weakness or indecision, being yourself intellectual and a good organizer with a strong sense of honor and duty. Unfortunately you hold on to too many old-fashioned ideas and are conventional, even austere. You waste time being too moody. You should gather Aquarius, Pisces, Taurus, Virgo, Scorpio, and Sagittarius, but not Aries, Cancer, or Libra.

## January 20 to February 18—AQUARIUS

Statistics show that most doctors and nurses are Aquarians. You love humanity and value peace very highly. You are unselfish and love change. You are always thinking new thoughts and trying constantly to improve anyone and everyone. You can be destructive, for you stir up conditions of discontent and dissatisfaction in your environment. You should associate with Pisces, Aries, Gemini, Libra, Sagittarius, and Capricorn. Taurus, Leo, and Scorpio are not for you.

## February 19 to March 20—PISCES

You have a dual personality, much like Gemini, which usually puzzles others and even yourself. You are dreamy, responsive, impressionable and sensitive, methodical and sympathetic. Yet sometimes you are too pessimistic and full of self-pity. You should try to develop a home—you're most comfortable at home. Surround yourself with Aries, Taurus, Cancer, Scorpio, Capricorn, and Aquarius. Be wary of Gemini, Virgo, and Sagittarius.

Well, did you find yourself in the above? Don't take it all too seriously, and don't split up with your mate after twenty years. My book might end up named as co-respondent.

Now we come to the boiling cauldrons and bat wings. No, I didn't say batmen, or batboys, or anything of that sort. Get out your high school Shakespeare and we'll start with the three ladies in the first scene of Macbeth.

Witches do exist. There are people who say I'm a witch, but witches aren't allowed to discuss those things, so my lips are sealed. I will say this, however: if you hint about it enough, your friends may become convinced of your powers. They'll think twice before crossing you.

Tea leaf reading, card reading, and palmistry are most helpful. Suppose you're at a party, and there's a handsome number there you want to be better acquainted with. What better way than to ask if you can read his cards, or his palm? Or suppose you haven't quite got the nerve to ask him. Fine, start reading anyone's cards, or have a friend who'll go along with you in staging a demonstration. It will earn you as much attention as setting fire to your hair and running naked through the room screaming, "Sanctuary!"—and takes far less effort.

Card reading, and the others, are like astrology, they open the door for conversations, and flatter him. And just think of the seeds you can plant in his innocent little mind. Be vague, and never predict anything too close to the present. If you say he's going to fall in love, you can make that immediate, and give a general description that comes close to your own. If you're predicting an accident, make that within a year or two. The odds are in your favor that way.

I can't go into all of the details of card reading here, but you can start with some basic details. Hearts signify love, diamonds mean money, clubs are trouble, and spades pertain to work. You take it from there.

As for the many areas of supernatural phenomena, I never treat them too lightly because I don't want to offend any spirits who may be looking over my shoulder. There are many unexplained mysteries, and I never fool with things I can't understand. But mark my words, the world of witches and fairies is close at hand. Wait until you meet a fairy, and then see if you still don't believe.

All right, I'll take away the crystal ball and pocket the silver coins. Let's get out of the cave and continue our journey. We're almost to the end.

# CHAPTER SIXTEEN
## LAUREL WREATHS
## AND WEDDINGS

THAT brings us very nearly to the finish line. I won, and you'll be adorned with the victor's wreaths—in this case, whatever particular goal you had in mind.

Much of what I've written has been included with the idea in mind that you wanted to marry and settle, at least for a while. Never mind what your friends tell you, even the best ones. Envy is a curious emotion, unfortunately common to even the nicest people from time to time. When they snicker over your dreams of a vine-covered cottage and other niceties, forgive them their little bit of maliciousness, and hold onto your dream. Pay no mind when they tell you that those things never work. Never is a very strong word—such relationships do sometimes work—for ten, fifteen, or twenty years.

Yours may be one of the right ones. It will be if you're willing to work, really work, every day. Never fall into the habit of thinking how long you've been together—treat each day as a new experience. Cruise him every time you see him, flirt with him, go into his arms each night as eagerly as though it were your first experience.

Don't expect him to know that you love him, tell him so, in word or deed. Put all the skill, seduction, beauty, and thought into keeping him that you utilized to get him, and he'll never stray far from you.

Of course, that's not to say that marriage is for you. Many people are in love with the idea of marriage. Others give themselves all kinds of reasons for needing or wanting a lover. Security is not really a reason for settling down with someone. Neither is the hope that it will make you more productive, or more successful. Nor should you marry because you're unhappy single— you'll only be unhappy married.

When you meet the one—the very one—with whom you know you want to live the rest of your lives, building together—that's the time to marry.

Until then, what are you fretting about? Being single is neither a crime nor a detriment. It can be a glorious, marvelous, fun-filled experience, rich in rewards. You're one of the people who do things, and to whom things happen. You're available, desirable, exciting and interesting. Enjoy it, live it to the fullest. When the time comes to give all that up, you'll know. Until then, I wouldn't worry about it, or pass by the goodies of life waiting for that man in white and shining armor to come bounding over the hill for you on his charger.

There's more, much more than I could put into any single book, that you can do for yourself, and to enrich your life. We're all unique, as I told you in the beginning. Not all of the rules I've applied will work as well for you. At the same time, there are qualities about you that are completely foreign to me, and that's as it should be.

All I've really tried to do is awaken you to the magic that already exists within you, to encourage you to make of yourself that wonderful creature you should and, I hope, will be. No matter what the raw material you have to work with, you can create someone exciting and desirable from it. Among some of the sexiest, most interesting people I know are some who had far less to work with than you.

There's the man I know with the drastically de-formed body, crippled for life. But with his mind he can more than compensate. There's another whose face, taken at surface value, would probably stop a clock, but beneath that homely exterior is a personality so warm and fascinating, I don't think anyone ever thinks about his physical limitations.

Some of them have been tall—one friend measures in over seven feet, and some of them as short as five feet. Some have been black, some yellow, and some every shade in between. But they've all had one thing in common—the ability to be themselves, and to make those selves as marvelous as possible. That's the goal I hope I've persuaded you to seek for yourself. I hope you will always be striving, never just content.

And now, having turned you into the ravishing thing you are, and set you loose, I've got to get busy. If I don't hurry, there'll be nothing left for me by the time you get finished.

# ABOUT THE AUTHOR

**V. J. BANIS** is the critically acclaimed author ("the master's touch in storytelling..."—*Publishers Weekly*) of more than 200 published books and numerous short stories in a career spanning nearly a half century. A native of Ohio and a longtime Californian, he lives and writes now in West Virginia's beautiful Blue Ridge.

You can visit him at http://www.vjbanis.com

www.ingramcontent.com/pod-product-compliance
Lightning Source LLC
Chambersburg PA
CBHW020000290326
41935CB00007B/242